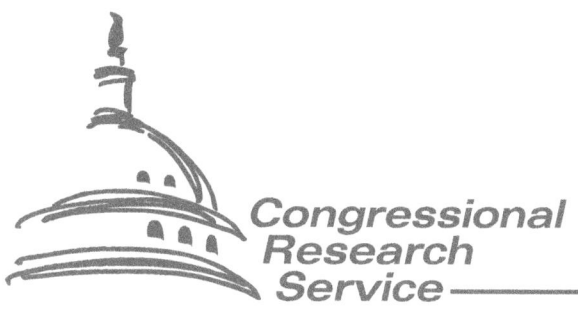

The Global Challenge of HIV/AIDS, Tuberculosis, and Malaria

Alexandra E. Kendall
Analyst in Global Health

February 23, 2012

Congressional Research Service
7-5700
www.crs.gov
R41802

CRS Report for Congress
Prepared for Members and Committees of Congress

Summary

The spread of human immunodeficiency virus/acquired immune deficiency syndrome (HIV/AIDS), tuberculosis (TB), and malaria across the world poses a major global health challenge. The international community has progressively recognized the humanitarian impact of these diseases, along with the threat they represent to economic development and international security. The United States has historically been a leader in the fight against HIV/AIDS, TB, and malaria; it is currently the largest single donor for global HIV/AIDS and has been central to the global response to TB and malaria. In its second session, the 112th Congress will likely consider HIV/AIDS, TB, and malaria programs during debate on and review of U.S.-supported global programs, U.S. foreign assistance spending levels, and foreign relations authorization bills.

Over the past decade, Congress has demonstrated bipartisan support for addressing HIV/AIDS, TB, and malaria worldwide, authorizing more than $52.5 billion for U.S. global efforts to combat the diseases from FY2001 through FY2012. During this time, Congress supported initiatives proposed by President George W. Bush, including the President's Emergency Plan for AIDS Relief (PEPFAR) and the President's Malaria Initiative (PMI), both of which have demonstrated robust U.S. engagement in global health. Through the Global Health Initiative (GHI), President Barack Obama has led efforts to coordinate U.S. global HIV/AIDS, TB, and malaria programs and create an efficient, long-term, and sustainable approach to combating these diseases.

In 2011, there were several significant scientific advancements in global health, including, most notably, evidence that early HIV treatment not only saves lives but can reduce the risk of transmission by 96%. Despite this scientific landmark, and ongoing progress in fighting HIV/AIDS, TB, and malaria, these diseases remain leading global causes of morbidity and mortality. Many health experts urge Congress to capitalize on recent gains and bolster U.S. leadership and funding to combat these diseases. In contrast, some Members of Congress have proposed cuts to these programs as part of deficit reduction efforts.

This report reviews the U.S. response to HIV/AIDS, TB, and malaria and discusses several issues Congress may consider as it debates spending levels and priority areas for related programs. The report includes analysis of:

- **Funding Trends:** Combined funding for the three diseases has increased significantly over the past decade, from approximately $832 million in FY2001 to $7.1 billion in FY2012. The bulk of the increase over time has been targeted toward HIV/AIDS, although in recent years funding for global HIV/AIDS has begun to level off. When compared to FY2011, funding in FY2012 included decreases for global HIV/AIDS, and slight increases for global TB and malaria programs. Some health experts applaud what they see as a shift toward less expensive efforts that maximize health impact. Other experts warn that divestment from HIV/AIDS could significantly endanger lives of those reliant on U.S. assistance and could reverse fragile gains made against the epidemic and other diseases.

- **Disease-Specific Issues:** HIV/AIDS, TB, and malaria each present unique challenges. Rising numbers of people in need of life-long HIV/AIDS treatment, as well as new evidence about the preventive benefits of early treatment, have heightened concern over the sustainability of treatment programs and incited debate over the appropriate balance of funding between antiretroviral treatment

(ART) and other HIV/AIDS interventions. Growing rates of HIV/TB co-infection and drug-resistant TB strains have increased calls for escalating TB control efforts. Finally, growing resistance to anti-malaria drugs and insecticides threatens malaria control efforts, leading to calls for more attention to reducing resistance and developing new anti-malaria commodities.

- **Cross-Cutting Issues:** Several cross-cutting issues are currently being debated, particularly in relation to increased efficiency and sustainability of HIV/AIDS, TB, and malaria programs under the GHI. These include
    - Health Systems Strengthening;
    - Country Ownership in Recipient Countries;
    - Research and Development;
    - Monitoring and Evaluation; and
    - Engagement with Multilateral Organizations.

For details on particular characteristics of the HIV/AIDS, TB, and malaria epidemics and the U.S. response, see the following CRS reports, by Alexandra E. Kendall.

- CRS Report R41645, *U.S. Response to the Global Threat of HIV/AIDS: Basic Facts*
- CRS Report R41643, *U.S. Response to the Global Threat of Tuberculosis: Basic Facts*
- CRS Report R41644, *U.S. Response to the Global Threat of Malaria: Basic Facts*

Contents

Introduction 1
Recent Developments 2
U.S. Policy Background 2
    Clinton Administration 2
    Bush Administration 3
    Obama Administration 5
U.S. Funding Levels and Trends 7
    Trends in Funding for HIV/AIDS, TB, and Malaria: FY2001-FY2012 9
    FY2012 Funding 11
    FY2013 Budget 12
Progress in Combating HIV/AIDS, TB, and Malaria 12
    Progress in Global HIV/AIDS 12
    Progress in Global TB 13
    Progress in Global Malaria 13
Key Disease-Specific Issues 14
    HIV/AIDS 14
    Tuberculosis 17
        HIV/TB Co-infection 17
        Drug-Resistant TB 18
    Malaria 19
        Drug and Insecticide Resistance 19
        Control, Elimination, and Eradication 20
Key Cross-Cutting Issues 22
    Health Systems Strengthening (HSS) 22
        Health Worker Shortages 24
    Country Ownership 26
    Research and Development (R&D) 27
    Monitoring and Evaluation (M&E) 29
    Engagement with Multilateral Organizations 31
Looking Forward 33

Figures

Figure 1. GHI Proposed Funding Distribution, FY2009-FY2014 6
Figure 2. Distribution of Funding for Global Health Programs, FY2001-FY2012 10
Figure 3. U.S. Funding Trend Line for HIV/AIDS, TB, and Malaria FY2001-FY2012 11
Figure 4. PEPFAR Funding for Prevention, Treatment, and Care FY2006-FY2009 15
Figure 5. Phases of Malaria Control Efforts, 2011 21
Figure 6. U.S. Bilateral and Multilateral HIV/AIDS, TB, and Malaria Funding, FY2012 32
Figure D-1. U.S. Bilateral HIV/AIDS Funding, by Country, FY2009 44
Figure D-2. HIV Prevalence Rates and PEPFAR COP Countries, 2009 45

Figure D-3. U.S. Bilateral TB Funding, by Country, FY2009 46
Figure D-4. TB Prevalence Rates and USAID TB Countries, 2009 47
Figure D-5. U.S. Bilateral Malaria Funding, by Country, FY2009 48
Figure D-6. Malaria Prevalence Rates and PMI Focus Countries, 2009 49

Tables

Table 1. U.S. Funding for Global HIV/AIDS, TB, and Malaria: FY2008-FY2013 8
Table 2. HIV/AIDS, TB, and Malaria Research and Development Funding, FY2008 28
Table C-1. FY2001-FY2013 Global HIV/AIDS, TB, and Malaria Funding, by Agency
  and Program 41
Table C-2. FY2001-FY2012 Global HIV/AIDS, TB, and Malaria Funding Totals in
  Constant Dollars 42

Appendixes

Appendix A. Acronyms and Abbreviations 36
Appendix B. HIV/AIDS, TB, and Malaria GHI Goals 38
Appendix C. HIV/AIDS, TB, and Malaria Funding 40
Appendix D. HIV/AIDS, Tuberculosis, and Malaria Program Maps 43

Contacts

Author Contact Information 50

Introduction

Human immunodeficiency virus/acquired immune deficiency syndrome (HIV/AIDS), tuberculosis (TB), and malaria are three of the world's leading causes of morbidity and mortality. Along with the direct health effects, HIV/AIDS, TB, and malaria have far-reaching socioeconomic consequences, posing what many analysts believe are threats to international development and security. Because of this, the United States has considered the fights against these three diseases to be important foreign policy priorities. In FY2011, of the $7.8 billion the United States spent on global health programs under the Global Health Initiative (GHI)—the Obama Administration's effort to coordinate and improve U.S. global health programming—approximately 83% was on bilateral and multilateral HIV/AIDS, TB, and malaria combined, with bilateral HIV/AIDS programs accounting for 63% of all funding. The United States is currently the single largest donor for global HIV/AIDS and has played a key role in generating a robust international response to TB and malaria.[1]

Despite growing international support for global health programs over the last decade and progress made in controlling HIV/AIDS, TB, and malaria in much of the world, significant obstacles remain in fighting the three diseases. In many countries, HIV infection rates are outpacing access to treatment, rates of drug resistance are increasing for TB and malaria, and health systems in resource-poor settings are under increasing pressure to address these diseases while struggling to provide basic health care.

Over the last few years, Congress has debated the U.S. strategy to confronting these diseases, including how to best support a long-term approach to these diseases that generates positive outcomes for global health in general. In response, implementing agencies have begun to make programmatic changes, and the Obama Administration has called for a revised U.S. approach to HIV/AIDS, TB, and malaria in the hopes of making related efforts more effective and efficient. This process has led to a broader discussion on how best to allocate global health funding, both within and between programs. The financial crisis and economic recession, and consequent calls to reduce the U.S. budget deficit, have led to decreased funding for these diseases in recent years, and have heightened the urgency of reevaluating U.S. global health investments. This report highlights some of the current challenges posed by HIV/AIDS, TB, and malaria, as well as several cross-cutting policy issues that the 112th Congress may consider as it determines U.S. global health funding for these three diseases, including

- Health Systems Strengthening,
- Country Ownership,
- Research and Development,
- Monitoring and Evaluation, and
- Engagement with Multilateral Organizations.

---

[1] For more information on the HIV/AIDS, TB, and malaria epidemics, and the U.S. response to each disease, see CRS Report R41645, *U.S. Response to the Global Threat of HIV/AIDS: Basic Facts*, by Alexandra E. Kendall; CRS Report R41643, *U.S. Response to the Global Threat of Tuberculosis: Basic Facts*, by Alexandra E. Kendall; and CRS Report R41644, *U.S. Response to the Global Threat of Malaria: Basic Facts*, by Alexandra E. Kendall.

Recent Developments

- In May 2011, results from a study demonstrated that early HIV treatment in couples with one infected partner reduced the risk of transmission by 96%.[2] This finding indicated the preventative benefits of HIV treatment and has been hailed by many as a "game-changer" in the fight against global HIV/AIDS.

- In November 2011, the Board of the Global Fund to Fight AIDS, Tuberculosis, and Malaria (Global Fund) announced that due to the current fiscal environment and resulting inadequate funding, it was canceling its 11th round of funding. While it has put a "transitional funding mechanism" in place to avoid disruption of existing services, it will not be offering any new funding until 2014.

- On December 23, 2011, the President signed into law the Consolidated Appropriations Act, 2012 (P.L. 112-74). Congress appropriated $7.3 billion for HIV/AIDS, TB, and malaria programs in FY2012, including slightly decreased or level funding for HIV/AIDS, and slightly increased funding for malaria and TB programs.

- On February 13, 2012, the President released the FY2013 budget request. The request included approximately $7.1 billion for HIV/AIDS, TB, and malaria programs, which included further decreases in funding for bilateral HIV/AIDS, TB, and malaria programs. At the same time, the request included a considerable increase in funding for the Global Fund. Despite the proposed decrease in bilateral HIV/AIDS funding, the budget request affirmed the Administration's commitment to treating 6 million HIV-positive people by the end of 2013, a target announced on World AIDS Day in 2011.

U.S. Policy Background

U.S. efforts to address HIV/AIDS, TB, and malaria have grown significantly over the last few decades, as successive Administrations and Congresses have increasingly recognized the severity and impact of these diseases.

Clinton Administration

An expansive U.S. government response to HIV/AIDS began under President Bill Clinton. In 1999, President Clinton launched the Leadership and Investment in Fighting an Epidemic (LIFE) Initiative to address HIV/AIDS in 14 African countries and India, marking the first interagency response to the epidemic. The following year, President Clinton signed into law the Global AIDS and Tuberculosis Relief Act of 2000 (P.L. 106-264), boosting funding for both HIV/AIDS and TB activities.

---

[2] Myron Cohen et al., "Antiretroviral treatment to prevent the sexual transmission of HIV-1: results from the HPTN 052 multinational randomized controlled trial," 6th International AIDS Society Conference on HIV Pathogenesis, Treatment and Prevention (IAS 2011), Rome, July 17-20, 2011.

Bush Administration

The George W. Bush Administration greatly elevated the fight against HIV/AIDS, TB, and malaria in the U.S. foreign policy agenda. In 2001, President Bush contributed the "founding pledge" to the Global Fund to Fight AIDS, Tuberculosis, and Malaria (Global Fund), a public-private financing mechanism for the global response to HIV/AIDS, TB, and malaria.[3] Shortly thereafter, in 2002, President Bush launched the International Mother and Child HIV Prevention Initiative, supporting prevention of mother-to-child transmission (PMTCT) activities in 12 African and 2 Caribbean countries.

In 2003, the Bush Administration announced the establishment of the President's Emergency Plan for AIDS Relief (PEPFAR), pledging $15 billion over the course of five years to combat HIV/AIDS, TB, and malaria. This pledge represented the largest commitment ever by a single nation toward an international health issue, and established a new and central role for donor governments in the fight against HIV/AIDS. Of the $15 billion, the President proposed spending $9 billion on HIV/AIDS prevention, treatment, and care services in 15 focus countries.[4] The President also proposed spending $5 billion of the funds on existing bilateral HIV/AIDS, TB, and malaria programs in roughly 100 other countries and $1 billion of the funds for U.S. contribution to the Global Fund.

The 108th Congress authorized the establishment of PEPFAR in May 2003 through the U.S. Leadership Against HIV/AIDS, TB, and Malaria Act of 2003 (Leadership Act, P.L. 108-25). The act authorized $15 billion for U.S. efforts to combat global HIV/AIDS, TB, and malaria from FY2004 through FY2008, including $1 billion for the Global Fund in FY2004. The act also authorized the creation of the Office of the Global AIDS Coordinator (OGAC) at the Department of State to oversee all U.S. global HIV/AIDS activities. Beyond increasing the scope of U.S. HIV/AIDS programs, the Leadership Act also shifted the focus of U.S. HIV/AIDS activities. In particular, while past U.S. global HIV/AIDS programs had primarily supported prevention activities, the Leadership Act set targets for extending anti-retroviral therapy (ART) and required that 55% of PEPFAR funds be spent on HIV/AIDS treatment.

Building on the success of PEPFAR in harnessing resources to combat a disease, President Bush announced the establishment of the President's Malaria Initiative (PMI) in 2005, which significantly increased U.S. funding for global malaria programs. PMI was a five-year, $1.2 billion commitment to halve the number of malaria-related deaths in 15 sub-Saharan African countries[5] by 2010 through the use of four proven techniques:

1. indoor residual spraying (IRS),
2. insecticide-treated bed nets (ITNs),

---

[3] For more information on the Global Fund, see CRS Report R41363, *The Global Fund to Fight AIDS, Tuberculosis, and Malaria: Issues for Congress and U.S. Contributions from FY2001 to the FY2012 Request*, by Tiaji Salaam-Blyther.

[4] The original PEPFAR focus countries included Botswana, Cote d'Ivoire, Ethiopia, Guyana, Haiti, Kenya, Mozambique, Namibia, Nigeria, Rwanda, South Africa, Tanzania, Uganda, and Zambia. Vietnam was added as a focus country in June 2004.

[5] The original 15 PMI focus countries were added over the course of three fiscal years. PMI began operations in Angola, Tanzania, and Uganda in FY2006, in Malawi, Mozambique, Rwanda, and Senegal in FY2007, and in Benin, Ethiopia, Ghana, Kenya, Liberia, Madagascar, Mali, and Zambia in FY2008. Nigeria and the Democratic Republic of the Congo were added as PMI focus countries in FY2011.

3. artemisinin-based combination therapies (ACTs) to treat malaria, and
4. intermittent preventative treatment for pregnant women (IPTp).

PMI represented a significant shift from past United States Agency for International Development (USAID) malaria programs. Until then, USAID's malaria programs provided primarily technical assistance. Under PMI, a minimum of 50% of the budget was devoted to the purchase and distribution of malaria-fighting commodities. The design of PMI also took into account some of the criticism levied against PEPFAR in its first two years, including the need to strengthen the alignment of programs with country priorities and better integrate programs into national health systems.

No analogous initiative was established for global TB. However, in 2007, the 110th Congress enacted the Consolidated Appropriations Act of 2008 (P.L. 110-161), which markedly increased funding for TB control efforts. The act provided unprecedented funding to expand USAID TB programs in high-burden countries. The act also recognized the growing threat of HIV/TB co-infection and directed OGAC to spend at least $150 million of its funds for PEPFAR on joint HIV/TB activities.

In July 2008, the 110th Congress enacted the Tom Lantos and Henry J. Hyde United States Global Leadership Against HIV/AIDS, Tuberculosis, and Malaria Reauthorization Act of 2008 (Lantos-Hyde Act, P.L. 110-293), authorizing $48 billion for bilateral and multilateral efforts to fight global HIV/AIDS, TB, and malaria from FY2009 through FY2013. Of the $48 billion, $4 billion was for bilateral TB programs, $5 billion was for bilateral malaria programs, and $2 billion was for U.S. contributions to the Global Fund in FY2009. The act also authorized the establishment of the Global Malaria Coordinator at USAID to oversee and coordinate all U.S. global malaria activities.

U.S. HIV/AIDS, TB, and malaria programs under the Bush Administration received strong bipartisan congressional support. At the same time, Congress and the global health community debated several aspects of PEPFAR, including

- the relationship between HIV/AIDS activities and other global health activities;
- the effectiveness of abstinence-only education;
- the integration of family planning into HIV/AIDS activities;
- the use of branded versus generic drugs;
- the role of recipient countries in setting assistance priorities; and
- the balance of funding between prevention, treatment, and care activities.

Many critics argued that PEPFAR was overly unilateral, relied too heavily on U.S.-based organizations, and did little to strengthen national health systems or country capacity to cope with the epidemic in the long run. The Lantos-Hyde Act was intended to respond to a number of these criticisms and support the transition of PEPFAR from an emergency plan to a sustainable, country-led program.[6]

---

[6] For an example of congressional discussion of these issues, see U.S. Congress, House Committee on Foreign Affairs, *PEPFAR Reauthorization: From Emergency to Sustainability*, 110th Cong., 1st sess., September 27, 2007, Serial No. 110-116 (Washington: GPO, 2007), http://internationalrelations.house.gov/110/37971.pdf.

Obama Administration

Partly in response to the above-mentioned debates, on May 5, 2009, President Barack Obama announced a six-year, $63 billion Global Health Initiative (GHI). The GHI is a comprehensive U.S. global health strategy that brings together a number of existing global health funding streams and programs managed by USAID and the Centers for Disease Control (CDC), as well as HIV/AIDS programs managed by the State Department and the Department of Defense (DOD). The initiative calls for the coordination and integration of established HIV/AIDS, TB, and malaria programs with one another and with other, broader health activities to maximize effectiveness, efficiency, and sustainability of U.S. global health programs. It also encourages increased efforts to strengthen underlying health systems and support country ownership. Finally, the GHI supports woman- and girl-centered approaches to global health, recognizing that women and girls often suffer disproportionately from poor health.[7]

HIV/AIDS, TB, and malaria programs are core components of GHI. The Obama Administration proposes spending 81% of all GHI funding on the three diseases from FY2009 through FY2014 (**Figure 1**). Since 2009, implementing agencies have produced multi-year HIV/AIDS, TB, and malaria strategies, which each articulate goals and strategies to support an integrated, long-term, and country-led approach to global health, in accordance with the GHI principles (see the "HIV/AIDS, TB, and Malaria GHI Goals" section). In a demonstration of his commitment to the fight against global HIV/AIDS, on World AIDS Day in 2011, President Obama announced an increased target of providing treatment to 6 million people infected with HIV by 2013.[8]

---

[7] *Implementation of the Global Health Initiative*, Consultation Document, USAID, http://www.usaid.gov/our_work/global_health/home/Publications/docs/ghi_consultation_document.pdf.

[8] The White House, "Remarks by the President on World AIDS Day," press release, December 1, 2011, http://www.whitehouse.gov/photos-and-video/video/2011/12/01/president-obama-world-aids-day#transcript.

Figure 1. GHI Proposed Funding Distribution, FY2009-FY2014
(U.S. billions)

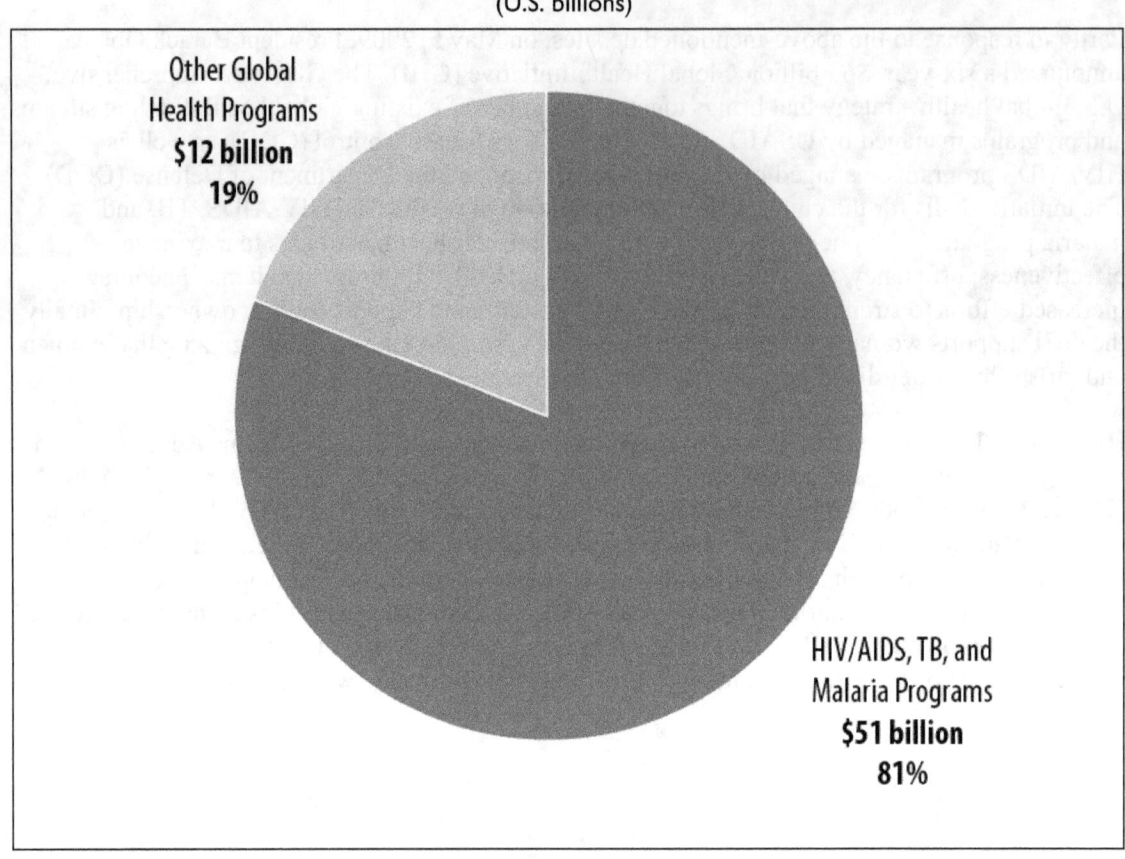

Source: CRS Analysis of GHI Consultation Document, *Implementation of the GHI*, February 2010.

In the three years since the launch of the GHI, the Administration has released a number of key documents demonstrating how the GHI principles are beginning to be implemented in the field. As of November 2011, 29 "GHI Plus" countries have been chosen to receive additional resources and technical assistance to accelerate implementation of the GHI and to serve as "learning laboratories" for best practices (the GHI will ultimately be implemented in every country receiving health assistance).[9]

In March 2011, the Administration released the "United States Government Global Health Initiative Strategy Document" as well as GHI Country Strategies outlining high-level priority areas and targets for country programs.[10] These multi-year strategies also serve as guidelines for new coordination efforts between PEPFAR, USAID, and CDC, as they aim to reduce duplication between programs, integrate services where appropriate, and better align programs with the priorities of partner governments. Several outside studies have documented early signs of progress toward a more cohesive and coordinated approach to global health, including in relation

---

[9] In July 2011, the first eight "GHI Plus" countries were named. They included Bangladesh, Ethiopia, Guatemala, Kenya, Mali, Malawi, Nepal, and Rwanda. In November 2011, a second round of 21 "GHI Plus" countries were named. They are Burundi, Democratic Republic of Congo, Georgia, Indonesia, Lesotho, Liberia, Sierra Leone, Tanzania, Ukraine, Vietnam, Botswana, Cambodia, Mozambique, Benin, South Africa, Namibia, Nigeria, Senegal, Dominican Republic, Philippines, and Swaziland.

[10] These resources are available at the Global Health Initiative website, http://www.ghi.gov/.

to HIV/AIDS, TB, and malaria programs.[11] Questions remain over how GHI will lend itself to significant innovation, whether early progress in coordination can be brought to scale, and whether efforts to better integrate global health activities can be sustained without significant additional resources. Also, despite the Administration's stated commitment to existing initiatives like PEPFAR and PMI, some experts have expressed concern that a new focus on coordination and integration will lead to decreasing support for touchstone disease-specific programs.

U.S. Funding Levels and Trends

Congress provides funds for HIV/AIDS, TB, and malaria assistance through several appropriations vehicles, including State and Foreign Operations; Labor, Health and Human Services, and Education; and the Department of Defense. Funds are appropriated to a number of U.S. agencies including the Department of State, USAID, CDC, and DOD. Congress also provides sufficient resources to the Office of AIDS Research at the National Institutes of Health (NIH) to support international HIV/AIDS research efforts. The agencies use the funds for bilateral HIV/AIDS, TB, and malaria programs and for contributions to multilateral organizations that address these diseases, including the Global Fund.

Since FY2001, U.S. funding in support of global HIV/AIDS, TB, and malaria programs has significantly increased. Funding for FY2012, as signed into law by the President on December 23, 2011, demonstrates continued congressional commitment to global HIV/AIDS, TB, and malaria programs, although it does not support the increased funding for these programs included in the President's FY2012 budget request. For a snapshot of recent years, **Table 1** includes U.S. actual, enacted, and requested funding for global HIV/AIDS, TB, and malaria from FY2008 through FY2013. **Appendix C** includes all U.S. actual and estimated funding for global HIV/AIDS, TB, and malaria from FY2001 through FY2012, as well as the President's FY2013 budget request.

---

[11] For example, see Center for Strategic and International Studies (CSIS), *The Global Health Initiative in Malawi: New Approaches and challenges to Reaching Women and Girls*, December 2011, http://csis.org/publication/global-health-initiative-malawi, CSIS, *On the Ground with the Global Health Initiative: Examining Progress and Challenges in Kenya*, March 2011, http://csis.org/publication/ground-global-health-initiative and Kaiser Family Foundation, *The U.S. Global Health Initiative: A Country Analysis*, February 2011, http://www.kff.org/globalhealth/8140.cfm.

Table 1. U.S. Funding for Global HIV/AIDS, TB, and Malaria: FY2008-FY2013

(current U.S. $ millions)

Agency or Program[a]	FY2008 Actual	FY2009 Actual	FY2010 Actual	FY2011 Actual	FY2012 Estimate	% Change FY2011 Actual – FY2012 Estimate	FY2013 Request	% Change FY2012 Estimate – FY2013 Request
USAID HIV/AIDS (GHCS/GHP)[b]	347.2	350.0	350.0	349.3	350.0	0.2%	330.0	-5.7%
USAID HIV/AIDS (Other Accounts)[c]	24.8	0.0	0.0	0.0	0.0	0.0%	0.0	0.0%
State HIV/AIDS	4,116.4	4,559.0	4,609.0	4,585.8	4,242.9	-7.5%	3,700.0	-12.8%
CDC HIV/AIDS	118.9	118.9	119.0	118.7	117.1	-1.3%	117.2	0.1%
NIH Global AIDS Research	411.7	451.7	485.6	375.7	364.5	-3.0%	388.9	6.7%
DOD HIV/AIDS	8.0	8.0	10.0	10.0	8.0	-20.0%	8.0	0.0%
FMF HIV/AIDS	1.0	0.0	0.0	0.0	0.0	0.0%	0.0	0.0%
HIV/AIDS Subtotal	5,028.0	5,487.6	5,573.6	5,439.5	5,082.5	-6.6%	4,544.1	-10.6%
USAID TB (GHCS/GHP)	148.0	162.5	225.0	224.6	236.0	5.1%	224.0	-5.1%
USAID TB (Other Accounts)	15.2	14.1	18.2	13.8	13.8	0.0%	8.0	-42.0%
TB Subtotal	163.2	176.6	243.2	238.4	249.8	4.8%	232.0	-7.1%
USAID Malaria (GHCS/GHP)	347.2	382.5	585.0	618.8	650.0	5.0%	619.0	-4.8%
USAID Malaria (Other Accounts)	2.4	2.5	0.0	0.0	0.0	0.0%	0.0	0.0%
CDC Malaria	8.7	9.4	9.4	9.4	9.3	-1.1%	9.4	1.1%
Malaria Subtotal	358.3	394.4	594.4	628.2	659.3	5.0%	628.4	-4.7%
USAID Global Fund Contribution	0.0	100.0	0.0	0.0	0.0	0.0%	0.0	0.0%
State Global Fund Contribution	545.5	600.0	750.0	748.5	1,300.0	73.7%	1650.0	26.9%

Agency or Program[a]	FY2008 Actual	FY2009 Actual	FY2010 Actual	FY2011 Actual	FY2012 Estimate	% Change FY2011 Actual – FY2012 Estimate	FY2013 Request	% Change FY2012 Estimate – FY2013 Request
HHS Global Fund Contribution	294.8	300.0	300.0	297.3	0.0	-100.0%	0.0	0.0%
Global Fund Subtotal	840.3	1,000.0	1,050.0	1,045.8	1,300.0	24.3%	1650.0	26.9%
HIV/AIDS, TB, and Malaria Total	**6,389.8**	**7,058.6**	**7,461.2**	**7,351.9**	**7,291.6**	**-0.8%**	**7,054.5**	**-3.3%**

Source: Compiled by CRS from appropriations legislation, congressional budget justifications, and the President's budget request.

Note: n/s = not specified.

a. Centers for Disease Control and Prevention (CDC); National Institutes of Health (NIH); Department of Labor (DOL); Department of Defense (DOD); Department of Health and Human Services (HHS), United States Agency for International Development (USAID), Foreign Military Financing Account (FMF).

b. Global Health and Child Survival Account (GHCS). In FY2013, the GHCS account was renamed the Global Health Programs (GHP) Account.

c. This includes funding from the Development Assistance Account (DA), the Economic Support Fund Account (ESF), and the Assistance for Europe, Eurasia, and Central Asia Account (AEECA).

Trends in Funding for HIV/AIDS, TB, and Malaria: FY2001-FY2012

Over the past decade, Congress has demonstrated significant support for U.S. programs targeting global HIV/AIDS, TB, and malaria. In particular, the enactment of the Leadership Act and the Lantos-Hyde Act raised the profile of HIV/AIDS, TB, and malaria and authorized increases in U.S. investments for countering each disease. Congress has also held a number of hearings in recent years to evaluate U.S. HIV/AIDS, TB, and malaria programs and to debate various approaches to fighting the diseases. While congressional action (including legislation and hearings) has tended to group the three diseases together, the response to each has varied widely, with HIV/AIDS receiving considerably more funding and attention than either TB or malaria.

Funding for each of the diseases has increased drastically since FY2001. Between FY2001 and FY2012, funding for bilateral HIV/AIDS, TB, and malaria programs in constant dollars has increased by approximately 600%, 201%, and 656%, respectively. Despite the marked increases in funding, particularly for global HIV/AIDS and malaria, there are significant differences in the percentage of the global health budget that each disease receives. Since the establishment of PEPFAR, HIV/AIDS programs have accounted for close to or over 50% of the global health budget, while TB programs have received between approximately 1.6% and 3.8%, and malaria programs have received between approximately 2.6% and 7.6% of global health funding, depending on the year (**Figure 2**). The establishment of PMI in 2005 raised the profile of U.S. global malaria programs, increasing its share of the global health budget from 2.8% in FY2005 to 7.6% in FY2012. U.S. support for fighting global TB has trailed that of HIV/AIDS and malaria and, unlike the other two, global TB has no U.S. presidential initiative or designated U.S. coordinator. Health experts continue to debate the appropriate apportionment of funding for the three diseases, including questions over the relative impact of and costs of treatment for each disease.

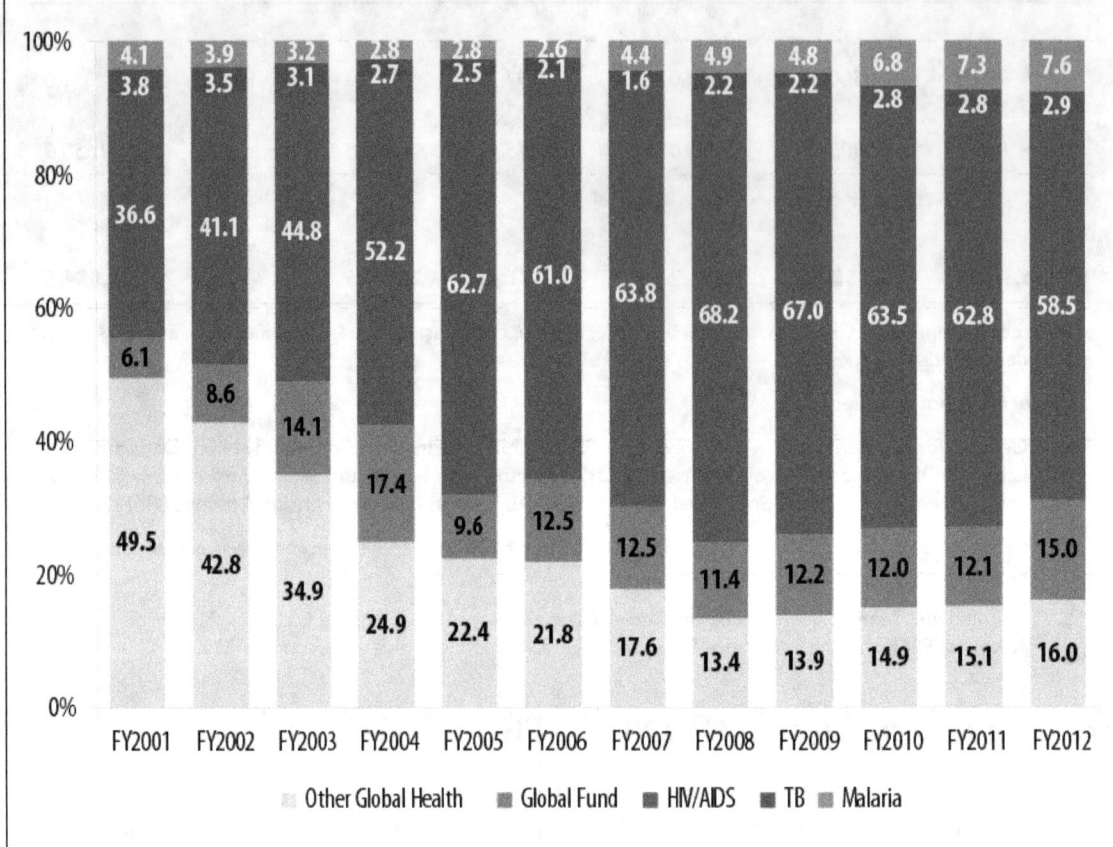

Figure 2. Distribution of Funding for Global Health Programs, FY2001-FY2012

Source: Compiled by CRS from appropriations legislation and congressional budget justifications.

Notes: "Other Global Health" includes programs targeting Maternal, Neonatal, and Child Health (MNCH), Family Planning/Reproductive Health (FP/RH), Neglected Tropical Diseases (NTDs), and other activities.

FY2001-FY2011 are actual funding amounts. FY2012 is an estimated funding amount.

Although absolute funding for all three diseases has increased since FY2001, specific trends for each disease have differed (**Figure 3**). Funding for HIV/AIDS increased rapidly from FY2004 through FY2008, during the first phase of PEPFAR, and has largely leveled off since the initiative was reauthorized. Funding for malaria increased significantly following the establishment of PMI in FY2006 and has since seen further increases. Funding for TB increased most rapidly in FY2008 and FY2010, followed by a slight decrease in FY2011 and a slight increase in FY2012.

Figure 3. U.S. Funding Trend Line for HIV/AIDS, TB, and Malaria FY2001-FY2012
(constant U.S. $ millions)

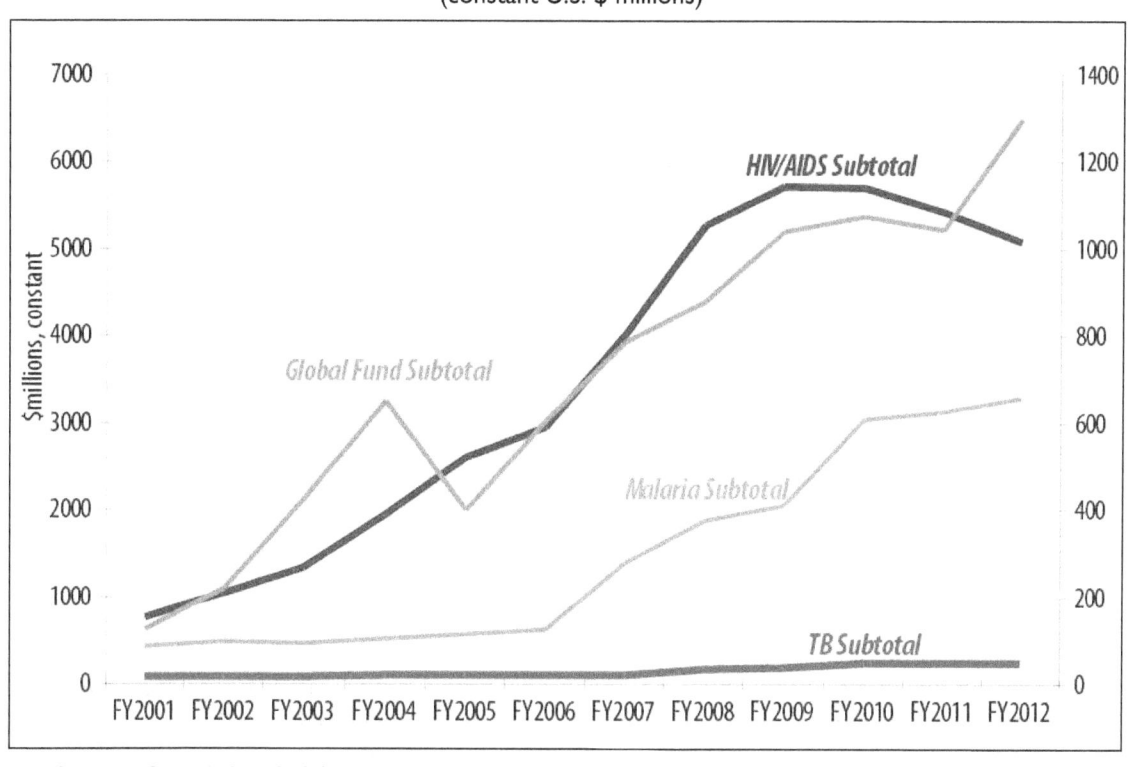

Source: Compiled by CRS from congressional budget justifications and appropriations legislation.

Notes: This graph has a secondary axis (in red) to account for the significant differences in funding amounts for HIV/AIDS and funding amounts for TB, malaria, the Global Fund.

FY2012 Funding

On December 23, 2011, the President signed into law the Consolidated Appropriations Act, 2012 (P.L. 112-74). The act included specific appropriations for State Department, USAID, HHS, and DOD global HIV/AIDS programs; USAID TB and malaria programs; and U.S. contributions to the Global Fund. While the estimated FY2012 funding level for all global health programs was higher than the FY2011 actual level, FY2012 funding for HIV/AIDS, TB, and malaria programs was slightly lower than in FY2011, and included a decrease in funding for global HIV/AIDS programs, a slight increase in funding for global TB program, and larger increases in funding for global malaria programs and the U.S. contribution to the Global Fund. Some health experts have expressed concern about the continuing flat-lining of global HIV/AIDS funding over the past few years. In particular, advocates have argued that any reductions in funding undermine recent scientific breakthroughs, which demonstrate that with adequate financial support, available prevention and treatment methods can be harnessed to significantly decrease new HIV infections and AIDS-related deaths. Others argue that given that HIV/AIDS funding tied to continuing lifelong treatment for people with HIV will likely be considered impervious, coupled with the new increased targets for treatment by 2013, the cuts made to HIV/AIDS programs may affect critical prevention and care activities, as well as broader HIV-related efforts in areas like health systems strengthening and country ownership.

While the FY2012 Consolidated Appropriations Act largely maintains support for programs targeting the three diseases, its enactment occurred after prolonged congressional debate over reducing the budget deficit through lower discretionary spending levels, with some Members proposing cuts to global HIV/AIDS, TB, and malaria programs. Some Members of Congress argued that these cuts could lead to important savings, while others strongly criticized any reduction in funding, arguing that it would undermine essential programs with humanitarian, development, diplomatic, and security implications. Compared to the President's request of $8.7 billion for all global health programs under the GHCS Account in FY2012, the House Subcommittee on State, Foreign Operations, and Related Programs mark-up of the FY2012 State-Foreign Operations appropriations bill recommended $7.1 billion for global health programs under the GHCS Account, representing an 18% decrease from the request, and the Senate Appropriations Committee-passed bill recommended $7.9 billion for global health, a 9.2% decrease from the request. The estimated total funding level for GHCS global health programs in FY2012 was higher than both the House and Senate recommendations, representing a 6.9% decrease from the Administration's request. A number of health advocates have applauded the relatively small reductions made in FY2012.

FY2013 Budget

On February 13, 2012, President Obama released the FY2013 budget request. When compared to FY2012 estimated funding levels, the budget requests funding decreases for all bilateral HIV/AIDS, TB, and malaria programs, including, most prominently, a 10.6% decrease in funding for bilateral HIV/AIDS programs. At the same time, the budget requested significantly increased funding for the Global Fund, representing a 26.9% increase in funding over FY2012 levels (see **Table 1**).

While the proposed increase in support to the Global Fund has been applauded by some health advocates, many express concern over the reduction in funding for bilateral programs, most especially PEPFAR programs. These experts argue that divestment in global HIV/AIDS and TB programs could imperil lives, reverse recent progress, undermine significant scientific findings, and lead to decreasing levels of support from other donors.

The Lantos-Hyde Act authorized $48 billion for global HIV/AIDS, TB, and malaria programs from FY2009 through FY2013, including contributions to the Global Fund. Current spending trends suggest that the authorized level may exceed appropriated amounts by over $10 billion.

Progress in Combating HIV/AIDS, TB, and Malaria

In late 2011, the World Health Organization (WHO) and the Joint United Nations Program on HIV/AIDS (UNAIDS) released new estimates of the scale of the global HIV/AIDS, TB, and malaria epidemics. The separate reports on each disease highlighted significant progress being made in the fight against the diseases, much of which is attributable to the leadership and support of the United States. The reports, characterized below, also identified major obstacles that remain.

Progress in Global HIV/AIDS

The 2011 WHO/UNAIDS report on global HIV/AIDS noted advancements in combating the global HIV/AIDS epidemic, including the landmark finding that among couples with one infected partner, early use of antiretroviral therapy can reduce transmission by at least 96%. The report also noted expanded access to several HIV/AIDS interventions, including HIV testing and counseling, anti-retroviral therapy, and drugs to prevent mother-to-child HIV transmission (PMTCT). Partly as a result of these interventions, both HIV-related mortality and incidence rates have declined.[12] In 2010, HIV-related deaths were close to one-fifth lower than in 2004 and the rate of new HIV infections was almost 25% lower than in 1996, the year that the HIV incidence rate is thought to have peaked. At the same time, WHO cited several ongoing challenges. HIV/AIDS is still without a cure or vaccine, and in 2010 alone, an estimated 2.7 million people were newly infected. New infections, combined with expanded access to ART for those already infected, create greater numbers of people requiring indefinite, lifelong treatment.[13]

Progress in Global TB

According to the 2011 WHO report on global TB, by 2008, most countries in the world had adopted WHO's Stop TB Strategy (the international guidance for prevention and treatment of TB). The global adoption of WHO prevention and treatment standards has enabled more than 55 million people infected with TB to receive treatment and prevented up to 7 million deaths between 1995 and 2010.[14] Global rates of new TB infection have been declining since 2002, and the absolute number of TB cases has been declining since 2006. The WHO report highlighted some ongoing obstacles to TB control as well. Progress in global TB control is also challenged by HIV/TB co-infection and new forms of drug resistant TB. Outdated tools for diagnosis and treatment, particularly in relation to HIV/TB co-infection and resistant forms of the disease, hamper further progress.[15]

Progress in Global Malaria

The 2011 WHO report on global malaria emphasized the effective scale-up of several malaria control interventions, including greater use of the latest malaria treatments, insecticide-treated bednets, indoor residual spraying, and drugs to reduce the transmission of malaria during pregnancy. Since 2000, 43 countries have experienced more than a 50% reduction in reported number of malaria cases and 8 African countries have experienced at least a 50% reduction in either confirmed malaria cases or malaria admissions and deaths. The decreases in each of these African countries are associated with intense malaria control activities. Despite this success, the report also noted obstacles in the fight against malaria. In particular, coverage rates of ITNs and IRS and access to ACTs remain low in many African countries, and increasing drug and insecticide resistance pose new challenges.[16] Finally, while WHO estimated that there were 0.7 million deaths from malaria in 2010, a study published in *The Lancet* in February 2012 estimated

---

[12] Incidence measures the number of people who contract a disease within a given time period (usually one year). Prevalence measures the number of people living with a disease at a given time.

[13] UNAIDS, *Global HIV/AIDS Response: Progress Report 2011*, 2011, http://www.unaids.org/en/media/unaids/contentassets/documents/unaidspublication/2011/20111130_UA_Report_en.pdf.

[14] World Health Organization (WHO), *Global Tuberculosis Control*, 2011, http://www.who.int/tb/publications/global_report/2011/gtbr11_full.pdf.

[15] Ibid.

[16] WHO, *World Malaria Report*, 2011, http://www.who.int/malaria/world_malaria_report_2011/9789241564403_eng.pdf.

that there were actually 1.1 million malaria deaths in 2010, indicating that the epidemic might have been far more severe than previously thought.[17]

Key Disease-Specific Issues

HIV/AIDS, TB, and malaria overlap geographically, share risk factors, and can worsen the symptoms of each other in instances of co-infection. Despite these common factors, each disease presents unique challenges, which Congress may consider as it debates the U.S. response to each disease. For more information on the particular characteristics of and U.S. response to each of the diseases, see the following CRS reports by Alexandra Kendall: CRS Report R41645, *U.S. Response to the Global Threat of HIV/AIDS: Basic Facts*; CRS Report R41643, *U.S. Response to the Global Threat of Tuberculosis: Basic Facts*; and CRS Report R41644, *U.S. Response to the Global Threat of Malaria: Basic Facts*.

HIV/AIDS

Sustaining the successes achieved in fighting HIV/AIDS presents new policy challenges. While AIDS-related mortality and HIV incidence rates have declined, improved access to anti-retroviral therapy (ART) combined with continued new infections has led to growing numbers of people living with HIV/AIDS and requiring lifelong treatment. At the same time, the new and long-term financial costs associated with expanded access to ART have increased concern over the sustainability of U.S. treatment programs, and have increased calls for considerable scale-up of prevention efforts.

The expansion of ART to treat HIV/AIDS has significantly reduced AIDS-related mortality. 2011 UNAIDS estimates suggest that 2.5 million deaths in low- and middle-income countries have been averted since the introduction of ART in 1995.[18] Treatment has been a central component of PEPFAR programs. According to a 2010 Government Accountability Office (GAO) report, from FY2006 to FY2009, 46% of PEPFAR funds were used to support treatment efforts, with the rest of the funds divided between prevention and care activities (**Figure 4**). As of September 2011, PEPFAR was directly supporting ART for over 3.9 million individuals in 30 countries—representing over half of the estimated 6.7 million people on treatment around the world.[19] In 2009, the Administration committed the United States to treating an additional 4 million people infected with HIV/AIDS from FY2009 to FY2014.[20] On World AIDS Day in December 2011, President Obama announced that the United States was committing to a new target of providing treatment to 6 million people by the end of 2013.[21]

---

[17] Christopher Murray et al., "Global Malaria Mortality Between 1980 and 2010: A Systematic Analysis," The Lancet, vol. 379, no. 9814 (February 4, 2010). WHO disputes these findings. For WHO's response, see Lisa Schlein, "WHO Stands by Its Numbers on Malaria Deaths," *Voice of America*, February 3, 2012.

[18] UNAIDS, *Global HIV/AIDS Response: Progress Report 2011*, 2011.

[19] Department of State, The United States President's Emergency Plan for AIDS Relief, *Using Science to Save Lives: Latest PEPFAR Results*, http://www.pepfar.gov/results/index.htm.

[20] The U.S. President's Emergency Plan for AIDS Relief: Five-Year Strategy, Annex: PEPFAR's Contributions to the Global Health Initiative, Office of the U.S. Global AIDS Coordinator, Department of State, December 2009, http://www.pepfar.gov/documents/organization/133437.pdf.

[21] The White House, "Remarks by the President on World AIDS Day," press release, December 1, 2011, http://www.whitehouse.gov/the-press-office/2011/12/01/remarks-president-world-aids-day.

Figure 4. PEPFAR Funding for Prevention, Treatment, and Care FY2006-FY2009

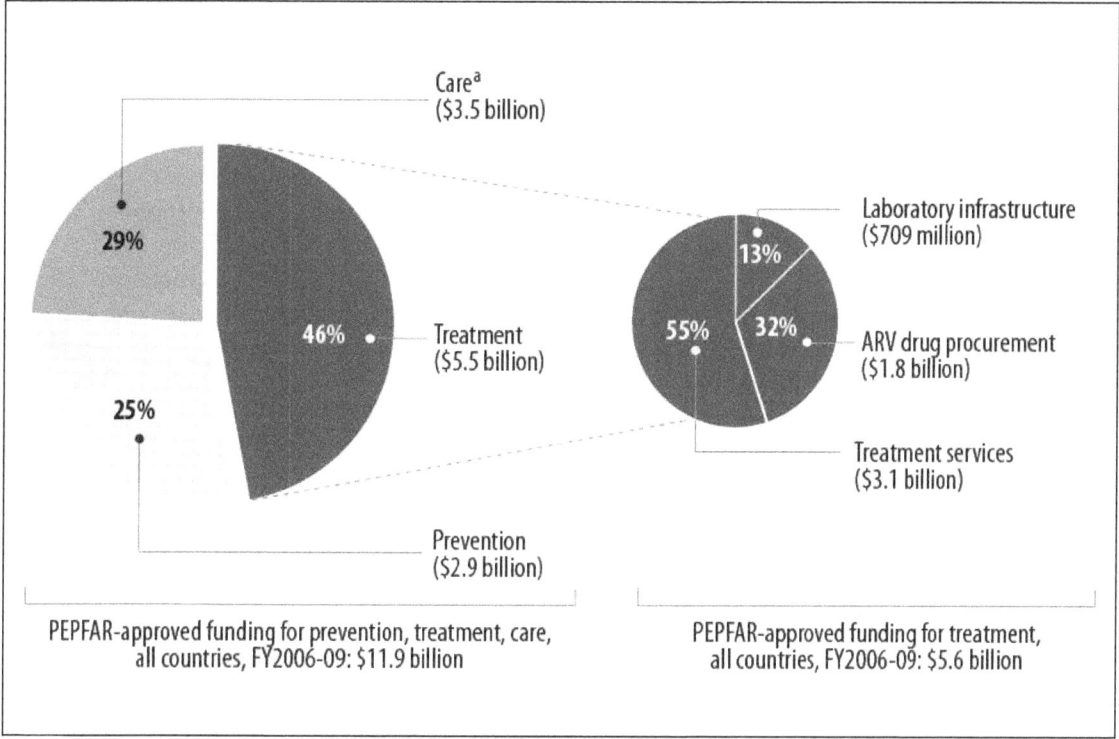

Source: GAO, *Global Health: Trends in U.S. Spending for Global HIV/AIDS and Other Health Assistance in Fiscal Years 2001-2008*, Report to Congressional Committees, GAO-11-64, October 2010, p. 8.

Notes: This graph refers only to FY2006-FY2009; it does not correspond to all PEPFAR funding since its establishment in 2004.

a. For FY2006 and FY2007, PEPFAR care program figures included funding for all pediatric AIDS programs, including treatment. In FY2008 and FY2009, PEPFAR counted pediatric care toward overall care funding and pediatric treatment toward overall treatment funding.

In spite of the strides made in HIV treatment, the number of individuals newly infected with HIV exceeded the number of individuals placed on treatment by almost a 2 to 1 margin in 2010. At the end of that year, the 6.7 million people receiving treatment represented 47% of those in need.[22] The number of people newly infected with HIV and requiring treatment is projected to grow significantly in coming years.[23] Expanding access to ART for new patients who will require lifelong treatment will increase long-term treatment costs.[24] Compounding this challenge is the potential for increased rates of drug resistance and consequent need for second-line therapies, which cost 5 to 10 times more than first-line drugs.[25]

---

[22] UNAIDS, *Global HIV/AIDS Response: Progress Report 2011*, 2011.

[23] Moreover, in July 2010, WHO published new guidance on ART for individuals in low-resource countries, advising that treatment begin at an earlier stage of illness, thereby increasing the number of people eligible for treatment.

[24] One model produced by *aids2031*, a UNAIDS-commissioned group of experts, estimated that total treatment costs would be between $11 billion and $18 billion per year in 2020. See, Aids2031, *Costs and Choices: Financing the Long-Term Fight Against AIDS*, Results for Development Institute, Costs and Financing Working Group, 2010.

[25] Anil Soni and Rajat Gupta, "Bridging the Resource Gap: Improving Value for Money in HIV/AIDS Treatment," *Health Affairs*, vol. 28, no. 6 (November 2009), pp. 1617-1628.

The logistical and fiscal challenges of scaling up treatment have led some experts to argue that prevention efforts must be rapidly scaled up so that HIV incidence can be reduced. In 2001, the results of an HIV prevention trial indicated that early initiation of ART in discordant couples[26] reduced HIV transmission by 96%, by lowering the viral loads of infected people and therefore reducing the possibility of transmission.[27] These findings have confirmed the preventative implications of HIV treatment and have reduced what was previously seen by some as a dichotomous choice between increasing funds for treatment versus increasing funds for prevention. At the same time, these findings raise new questions related to the appropriate distribution of limited—or decreasing—funding for global HIV/AIDS, including how funds should be divided between ART as treatment, ART as prevention, and other non-treatment-based forms of prevention. Some also argue that the United States must consider how to make more efficient use of available treatment resources, including in relation to earlier versus later initiation of treatment and the distribution of resources between first-line and second-line drugs.[28] The President's FY2013 budget request, which proposed decreased funding for bilateral global HIV/AIDS programs while also reaffirming the Administration's commitment to the new goal of treating 6 million HIV-positive individuals by 2013, demonstrated the importance of evaluating how to best allocate global HIV/AIDS funds.

Many HIV/AIDS experts stress that ART, as a tool of both treatment and prevention, must not only be used increasingly, but also in tandem with other increased support for "combination prevention" options, including biomedical, behavioral, and structural interventions (efforts to address the social, political, and economic factors impacting vulnerability to HIV).[29] In 2009, prevention-specific activities accounted for 22% of HIV/AIDS spending in low- and middle-income countries by all sources.[30] According to UNAIDS, several methods of prevention have demonstrated clear success. Prevention of mother-to-child transmission (PMTCT) has led to reductions in children infected with HIV, and male circumcision has led to reduced likelihood of uninfected men acquiring HIV from HIV-infected female partners.[31] At the same time, UNAIDS has argued that global prevention interventions are often not adequately directed at the populations most in need, including people who inject drugs, sex workers and their clients, and men who have sex with men (MSM).[32] A major factor limiting the success of ART-based prevention efforts, including early initiation of ART and PMTCT, is that more than 60% of people living with HIV are unaware of their HIV status.[33] Many experts argue that to improve the effectiveness of HIV prevention, there must also be efforts to expand HIV testing and counseling.

---

[26] An HIV-serodiscordant couple is one in which one partner is HIV-positive and the other HIV-negative.

[27] National Institutes of Health, National Institute of Allergy and Infectious Diseases, "Treating HIV-infected people with antiretrovirals protects partners from infection: Findings result from NIH-funded international study," press release, May 12, 2011, http://www.niaid.nih.gov/news/newsreleases/2011/Pages/HPTN052.aspx.

[28] Institute of Medicine (IOM), *Preparing for the Future of HIV/AIDS in Africa: A Shared Responsibility*, November 29, 2010, http://www.iom.edu/Reports/2010/Preparing-for-the-Future-of-HIVAIDS-in-Africa-A-Shared-Responsibility.aspx.

[29] See, for example, Carl Dieffenbach and Anthony Fauci, "Thirty Years of HIV and AIDS: Future Challenges and Opportunities," *Annals of Internal Medicine*, vol. 154, no. 11 (June 7, 2011); Reuben Granich et al., "ART in Prevention of HIV and TB: Update on Current Research Efforts," *Current HIV Research*, vol. 9, no. 6 (2011); and Mead Over, *Achieving an AIDS Transition: Preventing Infections to Sustain Treatment* (Washington, DC: Center for Global Development, 2011).

[30] UNAIDS, Report on the Global AIDS Epidemic, 2010, p. 63.

[31] Ibid.

[32] Ibid.

[33] Ibid.

In recent years, PEPFAR has placed new emphasis on prevention. For example, it committed to preventing more than 12 million new infections from FY2009 to FY2014.[34] PEPFAR's five-year strategy emphasizes scaling up combined interventions tailored to the key drivers of individual country epidemics, and puts particular emphasis on PMTCT and male circumcision activities. Despite this commitment, many health experts call for increased U.S. support of HIV/AIDS prevention efforts in general, and efforts targeting high-risk groups in particular. Many experts also urge the United States to increase its support for new methods to measure and evaluate infection trends and prevention program impact, in order to effectively tailor prevention programs to specific country epidemics and better assess the efficacy of various prevention programs.

While many Members of Congress agree that prevention must be a priority of HIV/AIDS programs, there is less congressional consensus over which prevention activities are most effective and should receive support.[35] In particular, some in Congress express reservation at U.S. support for prevention activities that they feel could be seen as supporting sex work or that may be integrated with family planning and reproductive health services that could be connected to abortion provision.[36] Many health experts argue that in order for prevention efforts to be successful, programs must be driven by data that indicate the needs of specific countries.[37]

Tuberculosis

Tuberculosis is the second-leading cause of infectious disease mortality around the world, following HIV/AIDS, yet it receives less funding than either HIV/AIDS or malaria. Gains in global TB control are challenged by growing occurrences of HIV/TB co-infection and drug-resistance, as both strain already-dated tools used for TB diagnosis, treatment, and surveillance.

HIV/TB Co-infection

TB is the leading cause of death for people with HIV. Of the 8.8 million new cases of TB in 2010, an estimated 1.1 million were HIV-positive. Along with HIV testing of TB patients, provision of HIV and TB treatment to those infected with both diseases, and general HIV prevention services for TB patients, WHO recommends three activities, known as the "Three I's," to address HIV/TB co-infection: the provision of a prophylaxis, known as Isoniazid Preventative Therapy (IPT), for HIV-positive people with latent TB; intensified case finding for active TB; and TB infection control for HIV-positive people. Some argue that WHO's "Three I's" have been unevenly applied

---

[34] The U.S. President's Emergency Plan for AIDS Relief: Five-Year Strategy, Annex: PEPFAR's Contributions to the Global Health Initiative.

[35] HIV prevention activities, particularly sex education, condom use, and interventions with sex workers, have been politically divisive in Congress. The Leadership Act recommended that 20% of HIV/AIDS funds be spent on prevention and required that 33% of prevention funds be spent on abstinence-until-marriage programs. A number of health experts argued that these spending directives limited PEPFAR's ability to address local prevention needs. The Lantos-Hyde Act removed the spending stipulations, but mandated that OGAC report to Congress should "activities promoting abstinence, delay of sexual debut, monogamy, fidelity, and partner reduction" amount to less than 50% of spending on programs aimed at reducing sexual transmission of HIV in countries with generalized epidemics.

[36] For more information on this issue, see CRS Report RL33250, *International Family Planning Programs: Issues for Congress*, by Luisa Blanchfield, and CRS Report R41360, *Abortion and Family Planning-Related Provisions in U.S. Foreign Assistance Law and Policy*, by Luisa Blanchfield.

[37] Lisa Carty, Philip Nieburg, and Suzanne Brundage, *Prevention of New HIV Infection: Priorities for U.S. Action*, Center for Strategic and International Studies, Washington, DC, January 2010, http://csis.org/publication/prevention-new-hiv-infections.

and that the global response to co-infection has been slow and uncoordinated, leading to limited access to diagnostic, prevention, and treatment services.[38] Compounding the uneven implementation of joint TB/HIV programming, WHO reports that among the 63 high TB/HIV burden countries, less than half reported treatment outcomes disaggregated by HIV status, making it difficult to assess the success of any existing programs.[39]

U.S. HIV/TB collaborative activities are coordinated and led by PEPFAR. In FY2008, Congress directed OGAC to provide at least $150 million for joint HIV/TB activities. As a result, PEPFAR has scaled up its HIV/TB activities in recent years, most notably with regards to HIV screening, testing, and counseling for TB patients.[40] Nonetheless, PEPFAR's FY2010 operational plan explains that integrating HIV and TB services remains challenging, in part due to operational differences between HIV and TB programs and programming that developed separately. Advocates of increased attention to HIV/TB co-infection argue that implementation of WHO's "Three I's" should be mandated as a core element of PEPFAR programming in settings with high co-infection rates. Similarly, while PEPFAR sets annual targets for HIV/TB activities for each focus country, some call for the creation of aggregate targets for joint HIV/TB activities.

Drug-Resistant TB

The past two decades have seen the emergence of multi-drug resistant (MDR) TB[41] and extensively drug resistant (XDR) TB.[42] Drug resistance primarily arises from poor treatment adherence or incorrect drug usage. In 2010, there were 650,000 cases of MDR-TB, and 58 countries had confirmed cases of XDR-TB.[43] In January 2012, India reported several cases of TB that seemed to be resistant to all available treatment.[44] Diagnosis and treatment of MDR/XDR-TB in low-resource countries has been limited,[45] due to shortages of sufficiently equipped laboratories and poor surveillance systems. Treatment for drug-resistant TB is more time-intensive and costly than for basic TB and many resource-poor countries are ill-equipped to adhere to WHO guidance that MDR-TB patients be treated in separate facilities from those with HIV. In the absence of a scaled-up response, MDR- and XDR-TB are expected to result in increased TB-related mortality rates.

The United States has begun to respond to the problem of mounting drug resistance, but there is not consensus over the extent to which U.S. programs should target these particular threats. Some

---

[38] Anthony D. Harries et al., "The HIV-associated Tuberculosis Epidemic—When Will We Act?," *The Lancet*, vol. 375 (May 29, 2010), pp. 1906-19.

[39] WHO, *Global Tuberculosis Control*, 2011.

[40] Advocacy to Control TB Internationally (ACTION), *Living With HIV, Dying of TB*, March 2009, http://c1280432.cdn.cloudfiles.rackspacecloud.com/ACTION-Report-Living-With-HIV,-Dying-of-TB-March-2009.pdf.

[41] MDR-TB is caused by bacteria that are resistant to at least two of the most effective anti-TB drugs. MDR-TB results from either primary infection with resistant bacteria or improper use of treatment.

[42] XDR-TB is caused by bacteria that are resistant to at least two of the most effective first-line treatments as well as any of the second-line anti-TB drugs.

[43] WHO, *Global Tuberculosis Control*, 2011.

[44] "Indian TB cases 'can't be cured'," *BBC*, January 17, 2012, pp. http://www.bbc.co.uk/news/health-16592199.

[45] According to WHO, in 2010 less than 5% of new and previously treated patients with TB were tested for MDR-TB. Likewise, the reported number of patients on treatment for MDR-TB represented only 16% of the estimated cases of MDR-TB among notified TB patients in 2010. See WHO, *Global Tuberculosis Control*, 2011, p. 2.

argue that in the absence of increased investment for drug-resistant TB interventions, MDR- and XDR-TB could become the dominant strains of the disease. Others argue that basic TB control efforts reduce the potential for drug-resistant TB, and that a shift in resources to MDR- and XDR-TB activities could threaten gains made in controlling basic TB.[46] A particular area of concern for TB advocates is a divergence in U.S. targets for TB and MDR-TB control between the Lantos-Hyde Act and the 2010 U.S. TB Strategy. While the Lantos-Hyde Act recommends that by 2013 the United States support treatment of 4.5 million TB cases and at least 90,000 new MDR-TB cases, the 2010 U.S. TB Strategy states that by 2014 the United States will support treatment of 2.6 million TB cases and 57,200 new MDR-TB cases. Advocates have urged Congress to support the fulfillment of the original Lantos-Hyde goals.

Malaria

Recent data suggest significant reductions in global malaria cases and deaths, due in part to anti-malaria efforts. However, new drug-resistant forms of malaria and insecticide-resistant mosquitoes threaten these gains. At the same time, the success in the control of global malaria to date has led policy makers to consider renewing efforts to eliminate and possibly even eradicate malaria, raising questions over the appropriate distribution of malaria funds.

Drug and Insecticide Resistance

Resistance to artemisinin-based malaria drugs—the most effective treatment currently available—has been identified in Asia, most prominently along the Thai-Cambodian border. Along with the challenge of drug resistance, 27 African countries and 41 countries worldwide have reported mosquito resistance to the insecticides used in Indoor Residual Spraying (IRS), and increasingly to the insecticide used in insecticide-treated bed nets (ITNs).[47] Factors leading to increased drug and insecticide resistance have included misdiagnosis of malaria, improper use of medications and insecticides, use of counterfeit malaria drugs, and lack of resistance surveillance.

Drug and insecticide resistance pose clear threats to U.S. malaria efforts, which support the use of artemisinin-based combination therapies to treat malaria, IRS, and ITNs. The United States has taken a number of steps to respond to drug and insecticide resistance. For example, the United States is working with WHO to monitor insecticide resistance and assist countries with the judicious use of insecticides, promoting a regular rotation of insecticides from different classes to reduce resistance to IRS, and supporting surveillance networks and drug resistance monitoring systems in Southeast Asia and the Americas.[48] Some experts call for an expanded commitment to reducing drug and insecticide resistance, particularly with regard to support for better surveillance systems. Others call for U.S. efforts to preemptively monitor for drug resistance in Africa.

---

[46] Lee B. Reichman, "Unsexy Tuberculosis," *The Lancet, Correspondence*, vol. 373 (January 3, 2009).

[47] Armel Djènontin, Joseph Chabi, and Thierry Baldet, et al., "Managing Insecticide Resistance in Malaria Vectors by Combining," *Malaria Journal*, vol. 8 (October 20, 2009), p. 233.

[48] President's Malaria Initiative, *Lantos-Hyde United States Government Malaria Strategy: 2009-2014*, April 25, 2010, http://www.fightingmalaria.gov/resources/reports/usg_strategy2009-2014.pdf.

Control, Elimination, and Eradication

In October 2007, the Bill and Melinda Gates Foundation issued a call for a renewed global commitment to the eradication of malaria.[49] Malaria eradication had been widely abandoned as a viable option in 1969, after a WHO-sponsored eradication campaign failed to gain traction in much of sub-Saharan Africa. Since the Gates announcement, key global health actors have compared and debated the merits and practicality of malaria control, elimination, and eradication efforts. The three levels of anti-malaria efforts can be classified as:

- **Malaria control:** reduction of the malaria disease burden to a level at which it no longer poses a major public health problem, with adequate surveillance and monitoring to address ongoing and emergent cases.

- **Malaria elimination:** interruption of local mosquito-to-human malaria transmission, and reduction to zero of new human cases in defined geographic areas, with continued measures to prevent reestablishment of transmission.

- **Malaria eradication:** permanent reduction to zero of worldwide malaria incidence, requiring no further public health action.[50]

WHO has categorized countries into the following malaria stages: control, pre-elimination, elimination, prevention of reintroduction, and malaria free (**Figure 5**). The United States and its WHO partners have endorsed the long-term goal of universal malaria eradication and are increasingly supporting elimination activities in eligible countries.[51] While the majority of PMI activities are focused in countries in the "control" stage, PMI has begun to support pre-elimination activities, such as intensified case detection and surveillance, in several specific areas within Zanzibar, Rwanda, and Senegal.[52] At the same time, PMI embraces the goal of malaria elimination in the Greater Mekong Region and the Amazon Basin by 2020, primarily through support for improved surveillance and monitoring systems.

Despite the widespread enthusiasm for eradication as a long-term objective, many health experts contend this goal is not feasible with existing malaria prevention and treatment tools, and will require new medications, prevention strategies, and a vaccine.[53] Many experts argue that malaria elimination presents a more realistic option, although some posit that a shift toward elimination activities may pose new challenges as well. For instance, some argue that over-emphasizing and investing in elimination activities in areas with fewer cases of malaria could divert funds away from basic malaria control in high burden countries.[54] Others argue that mass treatment in support of malaria elimination without the appropriate monitoring and surveillance capacity could lead to drug resistance. Finally, some warn that even if elimination is achieved, governments and donors must ensure that disease surveillance systems are in place to detect a resurgence of the disease.[55]

---

[49] Bill and Melinda Gates Foundation, *Malaria Forum*, October 17, 2007.

[50] WHO, *World Malaria Report*, 2010, p. 6.

[51] President's Malaria Initiative, *Lantos-Hyde United States Government Malaria Strategy: 2009-2014*, p. 5, 10.

[52] Personal correspondence with PMI Senior Policy Advisor.

[53] Leslie Roberts and Martin Enserink, "Did They Really Say ... Eradication?," *Science*, vol. 318 (2007), pp. 1544-5 and Marcel Tanner and Don de Savigny, *Malaria Eradication Back on the Table*, Bulletin of the WHO, 2007, p. 82.

[54] J. Lines, A. Schapire, and T. Smith, "Tackling Malaria Today," *British Medical Journal*, vol. 337 (2008), pp. 435-437.

[55] Richard Feachem, "Shrinking the Malaria Map: Progress and Prospects," *The Lancet*, October 29, 2010.

Figure 5. Phases of Malaria Control Efforts, 2011

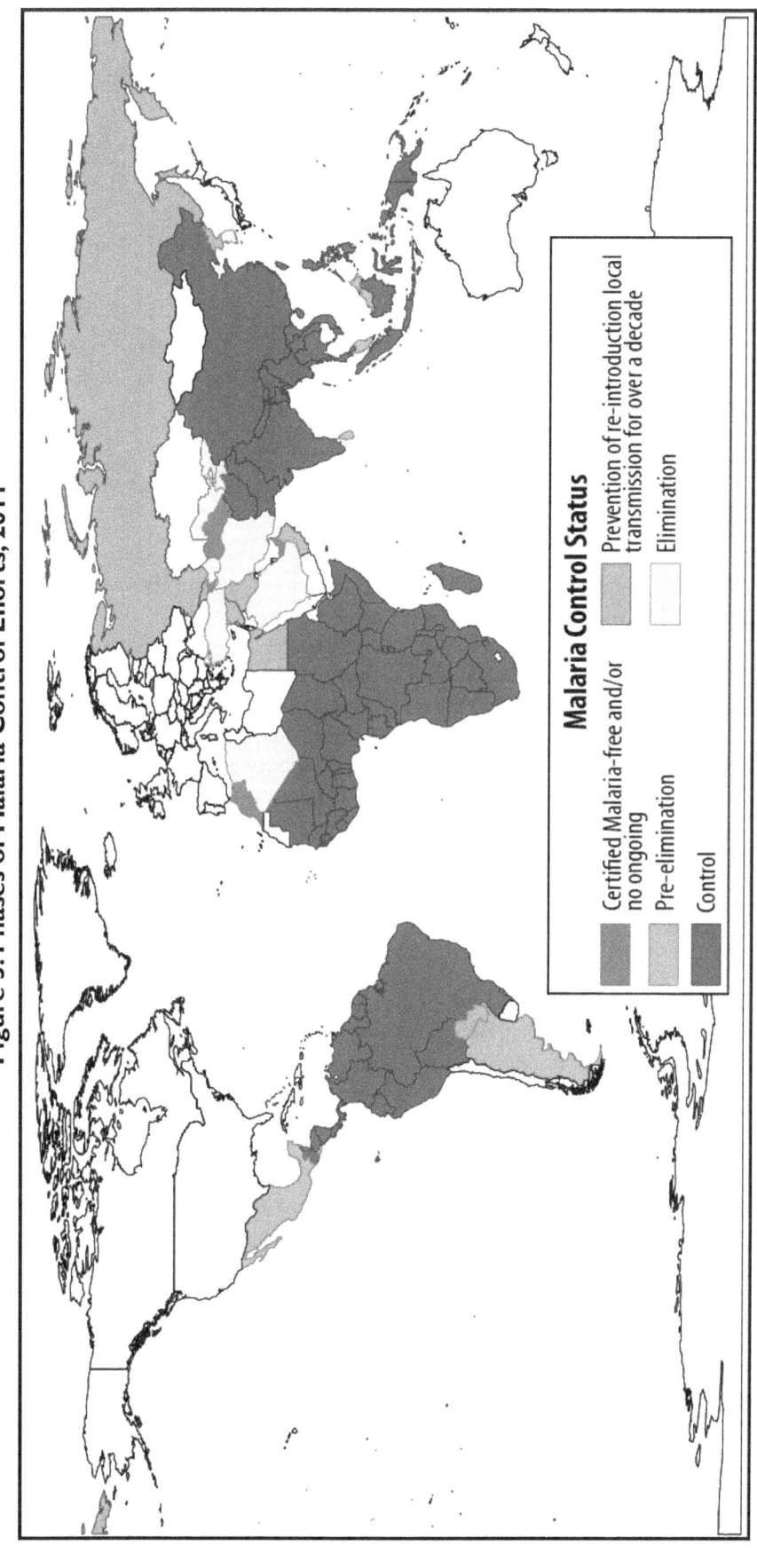

Source: WHO, *World Malaria Report*, 2011.

Key Cross-Cutting Issues

Along with the challenges specific to HIV/AIDS, TB, and malaria, a number of issues extend to all three diseases. This section looks at the following issues as they relate to all three of the diseases:

- health systems strengthening, including health worker shortages;
- country ownership;
- research and development;
- monitoring and evaluation; and
- engagement with multilateral organizations.

Health Systems Strengthening (HSS)

In recent years, weak health systems, including limited availability of health facilities, equipment, laboratories, and personnel, have been a critical obstacle to scaling up HIV/AIDS, TB, and malaria interventions. For example, shortages of ART have been reported in a number of African countries due to inadequate forecasting and information sharing systems.[56] Also, by 2010, only a handful of the 36 high-burden TB and MDR-TB countries had met the WHO recommendation of having at least one laboratory per 5 million people capable of culturing samples, the most definitive method for detecting TB.[57] USAID documents also cite inadequate clinical management and unavailability of drugs as common causes of fatality among hospitalized malaria patients.[58] These concerns have led many in the global health community to assert that health systems strengthening (HSS) must be considered an essential ingredient of a long-term approach to HIV/AIDS, TB, and malaria. HSS is one of the GHI target areas and has been integrated as a key goal in the U.S. HIV/AIDS, TB, and malaria strategies (**Appendix B**). At the same time, there is a lack of clarity over what HSS means and how it can be put into practice.

While there is widespread recognition of the need for stronger health systems, no international consensus exists on the operational definition of HSS. The clearest direction comes from WHO, which maintains that six "building blocks" are critical for a health system: service delivery, health workforce, health information systems, access to essential medicines, financing, and leadership/governance.[59] The GHI consultation document cites the following goals in the U.S. approach to HSS:

- Improve financial strategies that reduce financial barriers to health care (for example, increase government and/or private sector funding for health services);

---

[56] IOM, *Preparing for the Future of HIV/AIDS in Africa: A Shared Responsibility*.
[57] WHO, *Global Tuberculosis Control*, 2011, p. 56.
[58] USAID, *Global Health Initiative and the President's Malaria Initiative: Build sustainability through health systems strengthening*, 2009, http://www.fightingmalaria.gov/about/ghi/build.html.
[59] WHO, *Health Systems Topics*, http://www.who.int/healthsystems/topics/en/.

- Decrease disparities in health outcomes by providing essential health services, such as skilled birth attendance and voluntary family planning;

- Increase the number of trained health workers and community workers and ensure their appropriate use throughout the country; and

- Improve the health management, information, and pharmaceutical systems to reduce stock-outs.[60]

Despite identifying these components for HSS, the Administration has not yet identified specific indicators for meeting these goals. The GHI consultation document states that specific HSS targets will vary according to country-specific needs, demographics, epidemiology, and structural conditions (such as the socioeconomic and political environment). GHI agencies including the Department of State, USAID, and CDC are working on producing indicators for HSS; however, as of February 2012 these have not been released. While some applaud the plan to align HSS activities with individual country needs, others argue that in the absence of more precise targets and ways to measure impact, the concept of HSS has the potential to be more rhetoric than reality.[61]

PEPFAR, PMI, and USAID TB programs have been integrated into national health systems to varying degrees. Since its establishment, PEPFAR has been progressively integrated into national health systems, but it has also supported the establishment of many stand-alone systems and has funded a number of activities through international nongovernmental organizations (NGOs), rather than local networks (including government, private, faith-based, and NGO groups). For example, PEPFAR has supported country health information systems for some of its programs, but has also set up some of its own information systems to collect data. Similarly, while PEPFAR has used some national distribution systems for AIDS treatment, it has also financed its own supply chain systems to procure antiretrovirals in a number of countries.[62]

Given that PMI was established after PEPFAR, it was able to learn a number of lessons from PEPFAR's first few years in operation, including its relationship to the broad functioning of national health systems. As a result, PMI activities have historically been better integrated than PEPFAR into established clinics and laboratories. PMI services have also been frequently combined with other maternal and child health care services. Like PMI, USAID's TB programs have largely been integrated into general health services. USAID's TB programs are often implemented by local groups and USAID works closely with WHO TB initiatives to support the implementation of WHO's strategy for detection and treatment of TB known as "directly observed treatment, short-course for TB" (or DOTS), which emphasizes involvement of national governments in TB control.

Over the past several years, debate about the impact of single disease initiatives on health systems has intensified. Some have argued that U.S. single disease initiatives, particularly PEPFAR, have had a detrimental impact on national health systems. For example, some critics argue that such initiatives have led to duplicative planning, operations, and monitoring systems that have often

---

[60] *Implementation of the Global Health Initiative*, USAID, p. 13.

[61] Bruno Marchal, Anna Cavalli, and Guy Kegels, "Global Health Actors Claim To Support Health System Strengthening—Is This Reality or Rhetoric?," *PLoS Med*, vol. 6, no. 4 (2009).

[62] Nandini Oomman, Michael Bernstein, and Steven Rosenzweig, *Seizing the Opportunity on AIDS and Health Systems*, Center for Global Development, August 4, 2008, http://www.cgdev.org/content/publications/detail/16459/.

bypassed existing public institutions, doing little to strengthen country capacity.[63] Likewise, some maintain that single disease programs have usurped resources and personnel out of general health services, leading to reduced care in other health areas.[64] On the other hand, some argue that single disease initiatives have had a positive impact on broader systems. Advocates point to the role of HIV/AIDS, TB, and malaria funding in increased training of health care workers and improvements in health supply chain mechanisms, equipment, information systems, and health facilities.[65] Some experts further argue that the implied dichotomy between single disease programs and systems strengthening is a false one, and that support for one should not preclude support for the other.[66]

Health Worker Shortages

A particular challenge for health systems strengthening (HSS) is the shortage of health care workers in countries confronting HIV/AIDS, TB, and malaria. According to WHO, only 5 out of the 49 low-income countries meet its minimum recommendation of 2.3 doctors, nurses, and midwives per 1,000 people.[67] Sub-Saharan Africa, home to the majority of HIV/AIDS, malaria, and HIV/TB co-infection cases, boasts only 1.3% of the world's health workforce.[68] Shortage of health workers limits the number of HIV/AIDS, TB, and malaria patients that can receive testing, counseling, treatment, and care. Health worker shortages lessen the likelihood of proper diagnosis and supervision once a patient is receiving medication, increasing the potential for poor adherence and eventual drug resistance. The reasons for the limited workforce are myriad, but experts point to factors such as "brain drain"; chronic underinvestment in health workforces, including frozen recruitment and salaries; and work environments with few supplies and limited support.[69] Resource-poor countries with the highest disease burdens also suffer from widespread lack of educational and training opportunities.

In light of these challenges, U.S. HIV/AIDS, TB, and malaria programs have supported a range of efforts to build health worker capacity. Between FY2004 and FY2009, PEPFAR supported 5.2 million training and retraining encounters for health care workers.[70] These efforts have largely addressed health worker shortages through HIV/AIDS-specific training for existing health workers and "task-shifting" through which less technical tasks are transferred to others, including community health workers. In FY2009, USAID-funded programs provided training to an

---

[63] Roger England, "The Dangers of Disease Specific Aid Programmes," *British Medical Journal*, vol. 335, no. 565 (2007).

[64] Bunnan Men et al., "Key Issues Relating to Decentralisation at the Provincial Level of Health Management in Cambodia," *International Journal of Health Planning and Management*, vol. 20, no. 1 (January-March 2005), pp. 3-19.

[65] Jessica E. Price et al., "Integrating HIV Clinical Services into Primary Health Care in Rwanda: a Measure of Quantitative Effects," *AIDS Care*, vol. 21, no. 5 (2009), p. 608-614, and David Walton et al., "Integrated HIV Prevention and Care Strengthens Primary Health Care: Lessons from Rural Haiti," *Journal of Public Health Policy*, vol. 25, no. 2 (2004), pp. 137-158.

[66] Marco Vitoria, Reuben Granich, and Charles Gilks, et al., "The Global Fight Against HIV/AIDS, Tuberculosis, and Malaria: Current Status and Future Perspectives," *American Society for Clinical Pathology*, vol. 131 (2009), pp. 844-848.

[67] WHO web page on health workforces, *Achieving the Health Related MDGs: It Takes A Workforce!*, http://www.who.int/hrh/workforce_mdgs/en/index.html.

[68] Institute of Medicine, *Preparing for the Future of HIV/AIDS in Africa: A Shared Responsibility*.

[69] Ibid.

[70] OGAC, Celebrating Life: The U.S. President's Emergency Plan for AIDS Relief, Fifth Annual Report to Congress, 2009, p. 25.

estimated 63,000 health care works in DOTS and other TB interventions.[71] These efforts have included pre-service and in-service training on TB to health care professionals and training of community health workers. According to the U.S. TB Strategy, support is provided to health-related academic institutions in partner countries to ensure that TB is a standard component of health worker curriculum. In FY2010, PMI reported the training more than 36,000 health workers in the diagnosis and treatment of malaria with ACTs.[72] PMI programs sponsor malaria-specific trainings for health workers, particularly those working in maternal and child health, and for community health workers.

As with the general question of health systems strengthening, there has been debate over the impact of single disease initiatives, particularly PEPFAR, on the health workforce capacity. Critics argue that PEPFAR's role in workforce development has primarily benefited HIV/AIDS programs, with little impact on broader health systems. Moreover, observers maintain that in some countries compensation to health workers through PEPFAR programs has drawn staff away from other public health needs.[73] Several experts also assert that the short-term contractual agreements that PEPFAR programs often used to hire health workers can cause disruptions in treatment and care. Finally, some argue that the use of short-term contacts and "task-shifting" do not address the underlying constraints on creating a stable workforce.

In response to concerns about health worker shortages, the Lantos-Hyde Act recommends that PEPFAR support the training and retention of more than 140,000 new health workers by 2013. The act also specifies that these health workers should be trained to deliver primary health care rather than HIV/AIDS-specific skills. The GHI consultation document includes the goal of training 140,000 new workers through HIV/AIDS programs, but extends the time period to 2014. To meet this goal, PEPFAR launched the Medical Education Partnership Initiative (MEPI) and the Nursing Education Partnership Initiative (NEPI), which provides support through grants to foreign institutions in African countries to expand or enhance models of medical education.

Advocates applaud the new attention to health workers, although many argue that the United States should adopt a much higher goal for training new health workers if it is to adequately confront shortages. Some also argue that while the Lantos-Hyde goal of training new workers was directed specifically to PEPFAR programs, increased efforts by malaria and TB programs are also necessary, with the ultimate goal to train workers in broad-based primary health care skills. To this end, some experts argue that the United States should employ performance incentives for a variety of health service responsibilities, rather than just disease-specific ones. Some experts also urge the United States to increase steps to reduce the attrition and migration of health workers from resource-poor countries, such as through health workforce strategic planning, health workforce needs analysis, increases in health worker remuneration, and improvement to workplace policies.[74]

---

[71] USAID, *Building Partnerships to Control Tuberculosis, Fiscal Year 2009 Report to Congress*, October 2010, pdf.usaid.gov/pdf_docs/PDACQ888.pdf.

[72] PMI, *The President's Malaria Initiative, Fifth Annual Report*, April 2011, http://www.pmi.gov/resources/reports/pmi_annual_report11.pdf.

[73] Oomman, Bernstein, and Rozenzweig, *Seizing the Opportunity on AIDS and Health Systems*, p. 6.

[74] Paula O'Brien and Lawrence O. Gostin, "Health Worker Shortages and Inequalities: The Reform of United States Policy," *Global Health Governance*, vol. 2, no. 2 (Spring 2009).

Country Ownership

In recent years, the international community, including the United States, has placed growing emphasis on "country ownership" of HIV/AIDS, TB, and malaria programs. Country ownership refers to strengthening the capacity of recipient governments and local civil society to develop and manage their own health programs, including the ability to develop health plans, forecast monetary and infrastructural needs, and ensure financial support of programs. Congress has demonstrated its support for country ownership through several mechanisms, including the Lantos-Hyde Act, which called on the Administration to better harmonize U.S. HIV/AIDS, TB, and malaria efforts with the national health strategies of recipient countries. The Administration also includes country ownership among its seven GHI goals. Despite this, a number of concerns have been raised over the feasibility of this goal, including whether countries will be willing and able to progressively "own" U.S.-supported HIV/AIDS, TB, and malaria programs.

The Lantos-Hyde Act authorized PEPFAR programs to develop strategic agreements with national governments to promote host government commitment to and ownership of HIV/AIDS programs. Since enactment, PEPFAR has implemented "Partnership Frameworks" with a number of countries. Partnership Frameworks are nonbinding five-year joint strategic planning documents that outline the goals, objectives, and commitments of the U.S. and recipient government. Over the five years, the United States is expected to shift increasing portions of aid from direct service provision to technical assistance, with the goal of the recipient government assuming primary responsibility for the management and funding of the programs to the fullest extent possible. As of 2011, the United States has signed 21 PEPFAR partnership framework agreements.[75]

Unlike PEPFAR, PMI and USAID TB programs do not include a formal process of establishing agreements with recipient countries. Nevertheless, U.S. malaria and TB efforts have historically been better aligned with recipient country national plans than PEPFAR. According to PMI documents, malaria needs assessments and planning visits are carried out in conjunction with National Malaria Control Programs (NMCPs). Annual PMI Malaria Operational Plans directly support national malaria control strategies and PMI program targets are typically aligned with those of the host country. Likewise, U.S. TB support is generally provided to fill financing gaps identified in recipient country National Tuberculosis Plans (NTPs).

There is widespread support within the international community for countries assuming greater control over efforts to fight the three diseases. At the same time, a number of questions about the realization of this goal remain, particularly in relationship to HIV/AIDS. Some experts question whether recipient countries are in fact ready and willing to assume greater responsibility when few African countries spend 15% of their national budgets on health care, as they committed to do at the 2001 Abuja Summit.[76] Alternatively, some analysts doubt Congress will prefer to have recipient countries manage the substantial resources aimed at addressing these diseases, given the possibility that funds may not be spent as efficiently or effectively as possible, along with the

---

[75] PEPFAR website, *Partnering in the Fight Against HIV/AIDS*, April 2011, http://www.pepfar.gov/press/121652.htm.

[76] In April 2001, African Union (AU) Heads of States met in Abuja, Nigeria, for the "African Summit on HIV/AIDS, Tuberculosis, and Other Related Infectious Diseases." At the summit, African leaders signed the "Abuja Declaration on HIV/AIDS, Tuberculosis and Other Related Infectious Diseases," pledging to allocate at least 15% of their annual government budgets to their health sectors. This pledge was reiterated in May 2006 at a "Special Summit of the African Union on HIV and AIDS, Tuberculosis and Malaria," in Abuja, Nigeria.

potential for misuse of funds by government officials. The legally nonbinding nature of Partnership Frameworks has also led some to question how effective they are in practice.

A September 2010 Institute of Medicine (IOM) report focused on PEPFAR's country ownership efforts and found that activities were generally aligned with national HIV/AIDS strategies and helped to achieve national goals; however, the study raised a number of operational challenges to effective in-country management and control of global health programs."[77] Challenges included

- weak in-country capacity, including in technical expertise;
- significant U.S. funding for HIV/AIDS, TB, and malaria programs for international contractors and private organizations rather than recipient governments;
- indicators used by the United States to evaluate HIV/AIDS, TB, and malaria program performance often differed from those used by host countries; and
- limitations in PEPFAR's willingness to share information about its programs and funding with recipient governments.

Research and Development (R&D)

Research and development (R&D) of diagnostic, preventative, and treatment tools is a key component of any long-term response to HIV/AIDS, TB, and malaria. Currently, these diseases are the top three targets of funding for global health R&D and, together, account for close to three-quarters of all investments in global health R&D. In 2008, of all global funds spent on global health R&D, 34.9% went to HIV/AIDS, 15.1% to TB, and 18.3% to malaria. (**Table 2**).[78] The United States is the largest government donor for these efforts. Within the U.S. government, NIH leads a range of basic and clinical research activities on global HIV/AIDS, TB, and malaria, while CDC, USAID, and DOD each conduct field research related to these diseases. As the United States reforms its HIV/AIDS, TB, and malaria programs to better support sustainable approaches to health, spending levels for R&D and the areas of R&D priority are up for debate.

---

[77] U.S. Government Accountability Office (GAO), President's Emergency Plan for AIDS Relief: Efforts to Align Programs with Partner Countries' HIV/AIDS Strategies and Promote Partner Country Ownership, 10-836, September 2010, http://www.gao.gov/new.items/d10836.pdf.

[78] The George Institute for International Health, *Neglected Disease Research & Development: New Times, New Trends*, December 2009, http://www.ghtcoalition.org/files/gfinder_dec2009.pdf.

Table 2. HIV/AIDS, TB, and Malaria Research and Development Funding, FY2008

(current U.S. $ millions)

Disease	Total Global Funding	% of all R&D Investments	U.S. Funding[a]	U.S. Funding as % of Global Funding
HIV/AIDS	1,164.9	39.4%	736.1	63.2%
Tuberculosis	541.7	15.1%	128.2	28.2%
Malaria	445.9	18.3%	143.5	26.2%
All Diseases	2,956.0	n/a	1,258.3	42.6%

Source: The George Institute for International Health, *Neglected Disease Research & Development: New Times, New Trends*, December 2009.

a. This includes funding from NIH, USAID, CDC, and DOD.

Existing R&D investments in HIV/AIDS, TB, and malaria have led to some progress in the tools available to combat the three diseases, such as the development of simpler HIV/AIDS drug regimens and long-lasting insecticide-treated bed nets (LLINs) for malaria control. There have also been several important recent R&D accomplishments. In 2011, results from an HIV prevention study found that early use of ART in discordant couples led to a 96% reduction in HIV transmission.[79] A 2010 trial also demonstrated that HIV treatment used as prophylaxis reduced the risk of HIV infection by 44% in men who have sex with men.[80] Results from another 2010 study in South Africa, funded in part by the United States, showed that a microbicide gel was 39% effective in reducing a woman's risk of contracting HIV during sex.[81] In December 2010, WHO endorsed the rollout of a new rapid diagnostic test for TB and MDR-TB, funded in part by NIH. The test provides a diagnosis within 100 minutes, while existing tests can take as much as three months to produce results.[82] Finally, while no vaccine for malaria exists, research has been promising. There are currently over a dozen vaccine candidates in clinical development and one, produced by GlaxoSmithKline, is in clinical trial. If these are successful, the vaccine could be available as early as 2014.[83]

In many cases, however, the impact of these advances have been compromised by outdated or inadequate technologies. Despite progress made in AIDS treatment, even the most recent forms of ART include potentially severe side effects and many of the newer drugs, particularly second- and third-line therapies, are prohibitively expensive for many developing countries. Likewise, available HIV/AIDS treatment requires increased nutritional intake, which is often challenging for poor individuals and families. Many of the current TB diagnosis and treatment tools were

---

[79] National Institutes of Health, National Institute of Allergy and Infectious Diseases, "Treating HIV-infected people with antiretrovirals protects partners from infection: Findings result from NIH-funded international study," press release, May 12, 2011, http://www.niaid.nih.gov/news/newsreleases/2011/Pages/HPTN052.aspx.

[80] Robert M. Grant et al., "Preexposure Chemoprophylaxis for HIV Prevention in Men Who Have Sex With Men," *New England Journal of Medicine*, November 23, 2010.

[81] Quarraisha Abdool Karim, Salim S. Abdool Karim, and Janet A. Frochlich, "Effectiveness and Safety of Tenofovir Gel, an Antiretroviral Microbicide, for the Prevention of HIV Infection in Women," *Science*, vol. 329, no. 5996 (September 3, 2010), pp. 1168-1174.

[82] WHO, *WHO Endorses New Rapid Tuberculosis Test*, New Release, December 8, 2010, http://www.who.int/mediacentre/news/releases/2010/tb_test_20101208/en/.

[83] Rebecca Voelker, "As Trials Advance for a Malaria Vaccine, Policy Makers Urged to Plan for Its Use," *JAMA*, vol. 304, no. 21 (2010), p. 2348.

developed decades ago and have had uneven success. The most common method of TB diagnosis, sputum smear microscopy, is labor intensive and does not consistently detect TB. Also, current treatment regimens require people with active TB to take medicines for a period lasting 6 to 12 months and to be monitored during their entire treatment cycle. The emergence of drug-resistant forms of TB and malaria highlight the need for even more advanced diagnostic and treatment tools, appropriate for resource-poor environments. Treatment of MDR- and XDR-TB is considerably more expensive than basic TB treatment and can take up to two years, including significant time spent in a hospital with special facilities. Growing malaria drug and insecticide resistance threaten the success of the most effective available methods to control the disease.

Many health experts believe that U.S. funding for HIV/AIDS, TB, and malaria research and development lags behind what is needed. In particular, experts point to the need for increased R&D related to basic TB diagnostics and treatment, new drugs to tackle TB and malaria drug resistance, and an AIDS vaccine. Some argue that the long-term nature of R&D complicates efforts to raise financial support for the work, and the low incomes in the most affected countries provide little incentive for private companies to invest in expensive research. In recent years, the international community has taken some innovative steps to address this challenge. For example, in the absence of viable commercial markets for some health technologies for developing countries, a number of new nonprofit ventures, known as Product Development Partnerships (PDPs), have begun to support research and the development of drugs, vaccines, microbicides, and diagnostics. PDPs working on HIV/AIDS, TB, and malaria includes groups like the International AIDS Vaccine Initiative, the TB Alliance, and the Medicines for Malaria Venture. Similarly, in 2008, WHO supported the establishment of the African Network for Drugs and Diagnostics Innovation (ANDI), an initiative that aims to build Africa-based research capacity to respond to diseases on the continent. The United States is one of the largest public financiers for these efforts, but many experts advocate increased support of innovative approaches to R&D.

Many also argue that the United States should significantly increase its support for what is known as operations, or implementation, research. Operations research is the study of how technology is used in the field, and aims to identify factors that affect service delivery and impact implementation or scale-up of interventions. Advocates applaud the support for operational research in the GHI consultation document and argue that it should be seen as necessary for improving prevention and treatment outcomes and for addressing strategies in support of more sustainable HIV/AIDS, TB, and malaria programs.[84] The recent evidence in support of early use of ART as a prevention method has increased calls for innovative approaches to testing the impact, feasibility, and acceptability of this approach in the field.[85]

Monitoring and Evaluation (M&E)

In recent years calls have increased within the global health community for more monitoring and evaluation (M&E) to track health activities, determine progress in meeting targets, and evaluate the activities' impact on health outcomes. M&E is a key component of the GHI and is emphasized in the United States' HIV, TB, and malaria strategies (**Appendix B**). The United States has recognized the need to make its HIV/AIDS, TB, and malaria programs increasingly

---

[84] *Implementation of the Global Health Initiative*, Consultation Document, USAID, p. 8.

[85] Reuben Granich et al., "ART in Prevention of HIV and TB: Update on Current Research Efforts," *Current HIV Research*, vol. 9, no. 6 (December 2011).

results-based, yet these efforts remain nascent and experts have expressed a number of concerns over how to meet these goals for each of the diseases.

While a systematic, quantitative evaluation of PEPFAR's impact has not yet been published, the Lantos-Hyde Act mandated a comprehensive assessment of U.S. HIV/AIDS programs and their impact on health, to be submitted to Congress in 2012. In 2010, IOM released a consensus report outlining its strategic approach for conducting this evaluation. Congress has also required several targeted evaluations from GAO and IOM. In 2007, IOM conducted a short-term evaluation of PEPFAR, focusing largely on its ability to meet its outlined targets for delivery of prevention, treatment, and care services in its focus countries.[86] GAO has released reports in July 2011, analyzing PEPFAR's program planning and reporting processes,[87] and in September 2010, analyzing efforts to align PEPFAR programs with partner countries' HIV/AIDS strategies.[88] Neither the IOM nor the GAO evaluation included assessments of PEPFAR programs in relation to long-term health-related outcomes such as HIV incidence, prevalence, or mortality.[89] Congress has not mandated a systematic review of either PMI or USAID TB programs beyond annual reports that include progress on meeting predetermined targets. The U.S. malaria strategy indicates that a large external evaluation will be conducted and published in 2015 that assesses progress on all U.S. malaria activities undertaken through 2014.

The United States is taking steps to strengthen its ability to effectively monitor and evaluate its HIV/AIDS, TB, and malaria programs. In support of better M&E, PEPFAR has expanded its tracking of outcomes and impacts of its programs in the short and long term. In 2009, PEPFAR released its "Next Generation Indicators" (NGI), providing new indicators to track the impact of PEPFAR activities. Through this effort, PEPFAR has attempted to better align its indicators with those already used by many host nations and other international donors and to minimize PEPFAR-specific reporting, allowing country teams more flexibility to design M&E plans in line with national governments. NGI also includes new indicators related to program and population coverage as well as program quality. This marks a shift from past practices, in which M&E focused largely on program outputs, such as number of individuals on treatment.

Documents from the President's Malaria Initiative state that it is working closely with the Roll Back Malaria Monitoring and the Evaluation Reference Group to standardize data collection and use internationally accepted indicators of progress, and will assist recipient governments in conducting nationwide household surveys to measure changes in child mortality and malaria prevalence. Likewise, in support of TB-related M&E, USAID works with the WHO Global TB Monitoring and Surveillance project, the WHO body charged with leading TB M&E activities, to standardize TB control indicators. USAID TB programs also include efforts to bolster national M&E systems to track TB infection and mortality rates as a key component of DOTS.

---

[86] Institute of Medicine, *PEPFAR Implementation: Progress and Promise*, March 30, 2007, http://www.iom.edu/Reports/2007/PEPFAR-Implementation-Progress-and-Promise.aspx.

[87] U.S. Government Accountability Office, *President's Emergency Plan for AIDS Relief: Program Planning and Reporting*, 11-785, July 29, 2011, http://www.gao.gov/products/GAO-11-785.

[88] U.S. Government Accountability Office, President's Emergency Plan for AIDS Relief: Efforts to Align Programs with Partner Countries' HIV/AIDS Strategies and Promote Partner Country Ownership, 10-836, September 20, 2010, http://www.gao.gov/products/GAO-10-836.

[89] Eran Bendavid and Jayanta Bhattacharya, "PEPFAR in Africa: An Evaluation of Outcomes," *Annals of Internal Medicine* (April 6, 2009), http://www.ncbi.nlm.nih.gov/pmc/articles/PMC2892894/.

Despite these steps to strengthen U.S. capacity for M&E activities, a number of challenges remain. M&E requires collection of a variety of data from multiple sources, including household surveys, birth and death registration, census, and national surveillance systems. Resource-poor countries often have limited ability to produce data that is timely, standardized, and of a high enough quality to use for routine tracking and assessment of health programs. Malaria M&E efforts are particularly challenged because many resource-poor countries have weak health information systems necessary to track childhood health and many people infected with malaria, especially children, do not seek treatment in official health facilities. Similarly, gaps in TB coverage, treatment, and case detection impede effective and comprehensive M&E. Drug-resistant forms of TB pose new challenges to M&E efforts, as many resource-poor countries do not have the capacity to test for second-line drug resistance. Efforts to monitor and evaluate HIV/TB co-infection rates and activities are also precluded by limited information sharing between distinct TB and HIV programs.

U.S. M&E efforts are also challenged by the interaction in the field between U.S. global health programs and those of other donors, including the Global Fund and a range of private and NGO actors, which make it difficult to evaluate the outcomes of any one program. Finally, given the number of factors that influence the functioning and capacity of health systems and national governments, effective ways to measure the progress and impact of activities related to issues such as health systems strengthening and country ownership remain contentious. Indeed, PEPFAR has yet to develop specific indicators for measuring the effectiveness of activities related to HSS, country ownership, and HIV prevention.

Many have called for the United States to mandate regular and comprehensive M&E of its HIV/AIDS, TB, and malaria programs and increase support for in-country capacity to collect and assess health data. Some have also called on the United States to improve its data transparency and its dissemination of results to international and local partners. Experts have encouraged the alignment of health indicators used by the United States (through programs like PEPFAR and PMI) and those used by multilateral organizations and national governments. Some also urge the United States to support the use of national information systems for M&E as a way to strengthen these systems and increase country ownership of M&E. At the same time, other observers caution that additional measurement and reporting requirements have the potential to overburden already strained countries and programs and may reduce the time and money available for programs.

Engagement with Multilateral Organizations

The United States supports global HIV/AIDS, TB, and malaria efforts through bilateral programs as well as partnerships with and contributions to multilateral organizations. Over the last decade, Members of Congress have debated the appropriate balance between funding bilateral and multilateral global health efforts. This debate frequently focuses on the extent to which the United States should support the Global Fund to Fight AIDS, Tuberculosis, and Malaria (Global Fund), a multilateral public-private partnership established in 2002 to provide financial support for global responses to the three diseases.[90] The Global Fund estimates that in 2009 it provided approximately 21% of all funding for global HIV/AIDS, 65% of all funding for global TB, and

---

[90] For more information on the Global Fund, see CRS Report R41363, *The Global Fund to Fight AIDS, Tuberculosis, and Malaria: Issues for Congress and U.S. Contributions from FY2001 to the FY2012 Request*, by Tiaji Salaam-Blyther.

65% of all funding for global malaria.[91] Donors to the Global Fund include a number of governments as well as private and multilateral organizations. The United States is the single largest donor to the Global Fund, though U.S. bilateral spending on HIV/AIDS, TB, and malaria far outweighs contributions to the Global Fund and other multilateral groups (**Figure 6**).

Figure 6. U.S. Bilateral and Multilateral HIV/AIDS, TB, and Malaria Funding, FY2012

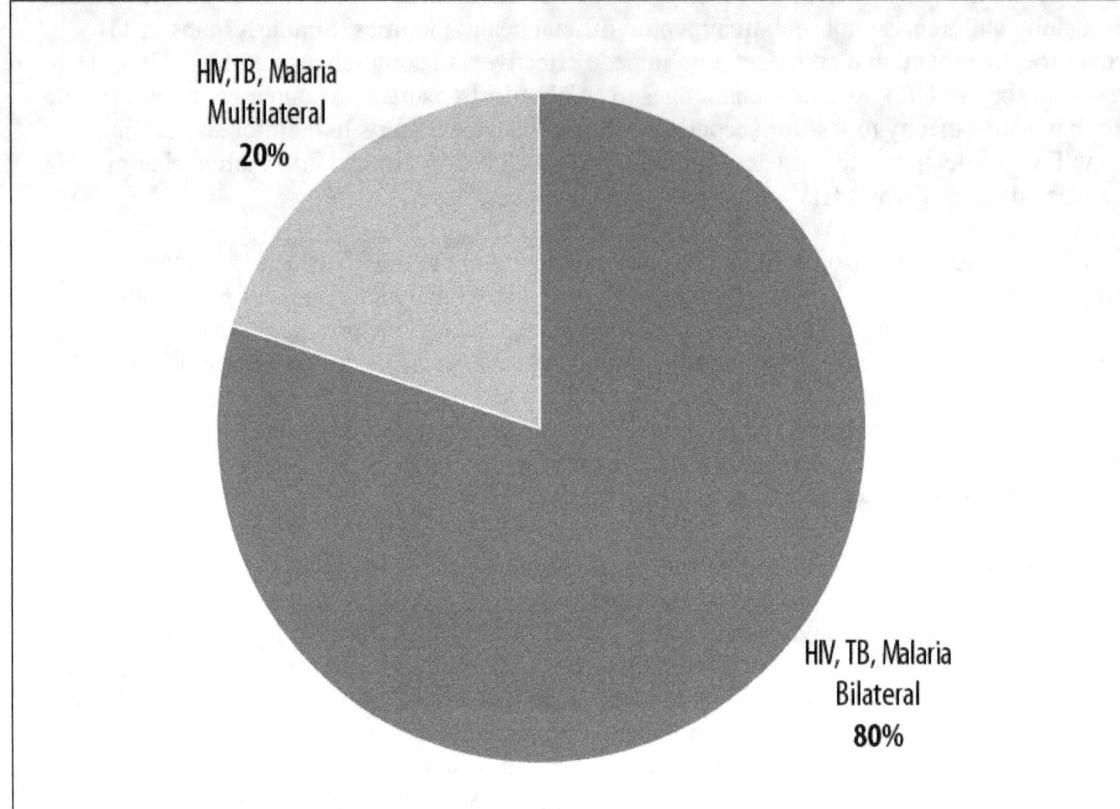

Source: Compiled by CRS from appropriations legislation and congressional budget justifications.

Notes: Multilateral Contributions include funding for the Global Fund, the International AIDS Vaccine Initiative (IAVI), UNAIDS, international microbicide research, and the Global TB Drug Facility. Contributions to the Global Fund make up the vast majority of investments in multilateral efforts. The United States also contributes to a range of other multilateral global health organizations, such as WHO, UNICEF, and the Global Alliance for Vaccines and Immunizations (GAVI), through non-HIV/AIDS, TB, or malaria specific appropriations.

The Obama Administration has indicated support for increased engagement with multilateral organizations, including the Global Fund. In October 2010, the President pledged $4 billion to the Global Fund over the course of three fiscal years—the first multi-year pledge to the Global Fund from the United States. While requesting decreased funding amounts for all bilateral HIV/AIDS, TB, and malaria programs, the FY2013 budget request includes a 27% increase in funding for the Global Fund over estimated FY2012 levels, fulfilling the President's multi-year pledge. The Administration has also emphasized nonfinancial ways in which the United States can support multilateral organizations, including better coordination in-country with multilateral

---

[91] The Global Fund to Fight AIDS, Tuberculosis, and Malaria, *Making a Difference: Global Fund Results Report*, 2011.

organizations, increased technical assistance to multilaterally funded field programs, and demonstrated leadership in shaping the policies of multilateral organizations (for instance, as a member of the Global Fund Board).

Despite this support, in November 2011, the Global Fund announced that due to limited resources available from donor countries, it would indefinitely postpone its 11th round of funding. In order to prevent any gaps in services, the Global Fund has instituted a "Transitional Funding Mechanism" (TFM), which will secure funding for programs facing disruptions in services currently supported by the Global Fund between 2012 and 2014. Documents released by the Global Fund have made clear that in this same time period, it will be unable to support any new interventions, nor will it support the scale-up of services, including provision of ART.

A number of experts contend that the Global Fund's decision demonstrates the critical need for increased multilateral funding from donors like the United States. Some argue that a reduction—or leveling—of funding to the Global Fund could imperil lives and cause significant losses in the progress made against the three diseases.[92] Some experts argue that the U.S. fight against the three diseases would be better waged through increased support to multilateral organizations rather than to bilateral programming. Specifically, advocates argue that multilaterals cede greater control of the programs to recipient countries, which supports the goal of country ownership. Some also argue that multilateral programs have more flexibility than bilateral programs, allowing them to better respond to locally defined needs. Likewise, some assert that funds are more effectively spent through multilateral mechanisms because donors can pool their resources and achieve economy of scale. Also, multilateral groups are capable of extending multi-year support. Some argue that this is particularly useful when addressing diseases that require long-term funding, like HIV/AIDS. Finally, some contend that U.S. engagement in multilateral organizations offers the United States opportunities to demonstrate its leadership in global health and encourage other countries to share in the global fight against the three diseases. As a result, some of these advocates applaud the President's decision to request significantly increased funding for the Global Fund in the FY2013 budget.[93]

Advocates of limited support for multilateral organizations argue that bilateral assistance increases the United States' ability to target health assistance to specific countries and determine funding priorities. In addition, others assert that bilateral assistance allows for better oversight of the use of funds by recipient governments and organizations. Some experts also contend that bilateral assistance is easier to track and measure than multilateral assistance, allowing for more effective monitoring and evaluation. Ongoing concerns about the capacity of multilateral groups like the Global Fund to detect and respond to corrupt practices propel this debate.

Looking Forward

The second session of the 112th Congress will likely exercise oversight of and debate the appropriate funding amounts for global HIV/AIDS, TB, and malaria programs and priority areas

---

[92] Doctors Without Borders, "As Global Fund Turns Ten, Lack of Political Support to Health Threatens Gains Against AIDS, TB, and Malaria," press release, January 30, 2012, http://www.doctorswithoutborders.org/press/release.cfm?id=5749&cat=press-release&ref=home-sidebar-right.

[93] For example, see Amanda Glassman, *GHI 2013 and the Rise of Multilateralism*, Center for Global Development, February 15, 2012, http://blogs.cgdev.org/globalhealth/2012/02/ghi-2013-and-the-rise-of-multilateralism.php.

within these programs. Discussions may focus on a number of critical disease-specific and cross-cutting issues, measurement of the effectiveness of the U.S. response, and tradeoffs the United States might consider as it sets priorities. As Congress reflects on these challenges, several overarching issues may also be considered:

- **Ways to assess impact and efficiency of global HIV/AIDS, TB, and malaria programs:** As Congress debates funding the fight against these three diseases, it will likely consider which methods to use in determining the distribution of finite global health and overall foreign assistance resources. The United States might face decisions over whether it should invest in the lowest-cost interventions, such as anti-malaria bednets, versus the higher-cost interventions that high-burden countries may be unable to afford, such as antiretroviral therapy. Similarly, the United States might consider whether it should support programs tackling the high-mortality issues, such as drug-resistant TB, or the more widespread and commonplace issues, such as malaria infection. The United States may also consider how it should balance its funding between high-impact activities, such as ART programs, with dramatic results and areas like health systems strengthening, which may yield few immediate results but which could result in significant long-term progress. More broadly, policymakers may weigh support for these programs against other foreign policy priorities.

- **Role of the United States in the global fight against HIV/AIDS, TB, and malaria:** The United States is a central leader in combating HIV/AIDS, TB, and malaria. Some Members of Congress have targeted global health funding for cuts as a way to reduce the U.S. deficit. Many supporters of these cuts have argued that the United States has played an overly generous role in combating issues like global HIV/AIDS, TB, and malaria, especially since these investments do not necessarily have direct implications for the wellbeing of U.S. citizens.

    Alternatively, many supporters argue that U.S. leadership in the fight against these diseases remains critical, particularly as new tools for treatment and prevention become available. Many of these advocates assert that given the prominence of the United States, any U.S. divestment could have significant negative consequences for some of the most vulnerable people in resource-poor countries. Some also point out that while the United States has been a key donor for HIV/AIDS, TB, and malaria, several European countries give more for these diseases as a share of their country's GDP. Finally, advocates assert that U.S. leadership is vital for sustaining the activities of the Global Fund, a key financial player in the fight against these diseases.

    Many advocates and critics of expanding U.S. global health assistance call for other countries, including a number of European countries, as well as emerging economies like China, India, Brazil, and Saudi Arabia, to begin playing a larger role in combating global HIV/AIDS, TB, and malaria. Advocates argue that increased efforts among other donors could help achieve the United Nations (U.N.) Millennium Development (MDG) goal "to combat HIV/AIDS, malaria, and other diseases," a goal which to which all U.N. member states have committed.[94] At the same time, there is disagreement over the ways in which U.S. leadership can and should motivate this kind of engagement.

---

[94] For more information on the Millennium Development Goals (MDGs) see the U.N. MDG website at (continued...)

- **HIV/AIDS, TB, and malaria assistance, economic development, and security:** Congressional consideration of U.S. HIV/AIDS, TB, and malaria programs may be affected by debate over their role in the broader U.S. foreign policy agenda. HIV/AIDS, TB, and malaria have undeniable humanitarian consequences. At the same time, many argue that these diseases also have important implications for economic development and security. Development experts argue that disease can threaten political and economic stability in fragile areas of the world, undermining U.S. interests abroad. Health experts believe that U.S. citizens are threatened by the spread of he infectious diseases across borders. Furthermore, foreign policy experts contend that global health efforts like PEPFAR have become critical diplomatic tools (often referred to as medical diplomacy) and have bolstered the image of the United States abroad, especially in sub-Saharan Africa. Alternatively, others caution against overly emphasizing the security and diplomatic implications of HIV/AIDS, TB, and malaria, and warn that doing so could lead to allocation of funding according to U.S. interests rather than human need.

(...continued)

http://www.un.org/millenniumgoals/aids.shtml.

Appendix A. Acronyms and Abbreviations

ACT	Artemisinin-Combination Therapy
AIDS	Acquired Immunodeficiency Syndrome
ART	Anti-Retroviral Therapy
CDC	Centers for Disease Control and Prevention
DOD	Department of Defense
DOTS	Directly Observed Treatment Short Course
FDC	Fixed Dose Combination
FP	Family Planning
GAO	Government Accountability Office
GHI	Global Health Initiative
Global Fund	Global Fund to Fight AIDS, Tuberculosis and Malaria
HHS	U.S. Department of Health and Human Services
HIV	Human Immunodeficiency Virus
HSS	Health Systems Strengthening
IOM	Institute of Medicine
IPT	Isoniazid Preventive Therapy
IPTp	Intermittent Preventive Treatment of Malaria During Pregnancy
ITNs	Insecticide-Treated Bednets
IRS	Indoor Residual Spraying
Lantos-Hyde Act	Tom Lantos and Henry Hyde United States Global Leadership Against HIV/AIDS, Tuberculosis, and Malaria Reauthorization Act of 2008 (P.L. 110-293)
Leadership Act	U.S. Leadership Against HIV/AIDS, Tuberculosis, and Malaria Act of 2003 (P.L. 108-25)
LIFE Initiative	Leadership and Investment in Fighting an Epidemic Initiative
LLINs	Long-Lasting Insecticidal Nets
M&E	Monitoring and Evaluation
MDR-TB	Multidrug-resistant Tuberculosis
MEPI	Medical Education Partnership Initiative
MNCH	Maternal, Newborn, and Child health
MSM	Men who Have Sex with Men
NEPI	Nursing Education Partnership Initiative
NIH	National Institutes of Health
NMCP	National Malaria Control Program
NTD	Neglected Tropical Disease
NTP	National Tuberculosis Plan
OGAC	Office of the Global AIDS Coordinator, Department of State
PEPFAR	President's Emergency Plan for AIDS Relief
PMI	President's Malaria Initiative

PMTCT	Prevention of Mother-to-Child Transmission
R&D	Research and Development
RH	Reproductive Health
TB	Tuberculosis
U.N.	United Nations
UNAIDS	Joint United Nations Program on HIV/AIDS
USAID	U.S. Agency for International Development
WHO	World Health Organization
XDR-TB	Extensively Drug-Resistant Tuberculosis

Appendix B. HIV/AIDS, TB, and Malaria GHI Goals

PEPFAR Strategy Targets

GHI set a number of goals to be reached from FY2010 through FY2014. GHI goals and projected targets for PEPFAR are:[95]

- provide direct support for more than four million people on treatment;[96]
- support the prevention of more than 12 million new HIV infections;
- ensure that every partner country with a generalized HIV epidemic has both 80% coverage of testing for pregnant women at the national level, and 85% coverage of antiretroviral drug prophylaxis and treatment as indicated, of women found to be HIV-infected;
- double the number of at-risk babies born HIV-free, from a baseline of 240,000 babies of HIV-positive mothers born HIV-negative during the first five years of PEPFAR;
- provide direct support for care for more than 12 million people, including 5 million orphans and vulnerable children;
- support training and retention of more than 140,000 new health care workers to strengthen health systems; and
- ensure that in each country with major PEPFAR investment, the partner government leads efforts to evaluate and define needs and roles in the national response.

U.S. TB Strategy Targets

GHI goals and projected targets for U.S. TB programs are:[97]

- to contribute to a 50% reduction in TB deaths and disease burden from the 1990 baseline;
- to sustain or exceed the detection of at least 70% of sputum smear-positive cases of TB and successfully treat at least 85% of cases detected in countries with established USG tuberculosis programs;
- to successfully treat 2.6 million new sputum smear-positive TB patients under DOTS programs by 2014, primarily through support for need services,

---

[95] The U.S. President's Emergency Plan for AIDS Relief: Five-Year Strategy, Annex: PEPFAR's Contributions to the Global Health Initiative, Office of the U.S. Global AIDS Coordinator, Department of State, December 2009, http://www.pepfar.gov/documents/organization/133437.pdf.

[96] On World AIDS Day 2011, President Obama announced an increased goal of treating 6 million people by 2013.

[97] USAID, et al., *Lantos-Hyde United States Government Tuberculosis Strategy, 2009-2014*, March 24, 2010, http://www.usaid.gov/our_work/global_health/id/tuberculosis/publications/usg-tb_strategy2010.pdf.

commodities, health workers, and training, and additional treatment through coordinated multilateral efforts; and

- to diagnose and initiate treatment of at least 57,2000 new MDR-TB cases by 2014 and providing additional treatment through coordinated multilateral efforts.

U.S. Malaria Strategy Targets

GHI goals and projected targets for U.S. malaria programs are:[98]

- to achieve Africa-wide impact, by halving the burden of malaria (morbidity and mortality) in 70% of at-risk populations in sub-Saharan Africa (approximately 450 million people), thereby removing malaria as a major public health problem and promoting economic growth and development throughout the region;

- to limit the spread of anti-malaria multi-drug resistance in Southeast Asia and the Americas;

- to increase emphasis on strategic integration of malaria prevention and treatment activities with maternal and child health, HIV/AIDS, neglected tropical diseases, and tuberculosis programs, and on multilateral collaboration to achieve internationally accepted goals;

- to intensify present efforts to strengthen health systems and strengthen the capacity of host-country workforces to ensure sustainability;

- to assist host countries to revise and update their National Malaria Control Strategies and Plans to reflect the declining burden of malaria, and link programming of U.S. malaria control resources to those host country strategies; and

- to ensure a woman-centered approach for malaria prevention and treatment activities at both the community and health facility levels, since women are the primary caretakers of young children in most families and are in the best position to help promote health behaviors related to malaria.

---

[98] USAID, *Lantos-Hyde United States Government Malaria Strategy, 2009-2014*, April 25, 2010, http://www.fightingmalaria.gov/resources/reports/usg_strategy2009-2014.pdf.

Appendix C. HIV/AIDS, TB, and Malaria Funding

Table C-1 presents an overview of U.S. funding for global HIV/AIDS, TB, and malaria efforts. The table does not include global health spending that does not correlate to specific congressional appropriations. For instance, CDC does not receive appropriations for global TB programs specifically, but spends a portion of its overall TB budget on international programs. Along with CDC global TB spending, the table does not include data for NIH and DOD malaria research.

Table C-2 presents the total amounts of U.S. funding for global HIV/AIDS, TB, and malaria efforts in constant dollars.

Table C-1. FY2001-FY2013 Global HIV/AIDS, TB, and Malaria Funding, by Agency and Program
(current U.S. $ millions)

Agency/Program[a]	FY2001 Actual	FY2002 Actual	FY2003 Actual	FY2004 Actual	FY2005 Actual	FY2006 Actual	FY2007 Actual	FY2008 Actual	FY2009 Actual	FY2010 Actual	FY2011 Actual	FY2012 Estimate	FY2013 Request
USAID HIV/AIDS (CSH/GHCS/GHP)	305.0	395.0	587.7	513.5	347.2	346.5	325.0	347.2	350.0	350.0	349.3	350.0	330.0
USAID HIV/AIDS (Other[b])	13.0	29.0	35.8	42.0	37.5	27.3	20.9	24.8	0.0	0.0	0.0	0.0	0.0
State HIV/AIDS (GHAI/GHCS/GHP)	n/a	n/a	n/a	488.1	1373.9	1777.1	2869.0	4116.4	4559.0	4609.0	4585.8	4242.9	3700.0
CDC HIV/AIDS	104.5	168.7	182.6	266.9	123.8	122.6	121.0	118.9	118.9	119.0	118.7	117.1	117.2
NIH AIDS Research	160.1	218.2	278.5	317.2	369.5	373.0	361.7	411.7	451.7	485.6	375.7	364.5	388.9
DOL HIV/AIDS	10.0	10.0	9.9	9.9	2.0	0.0	0.0	0.0	0.0	0.0	0.0	0.0	0.0
DOD HIV/AIDS	10.0	14.0	7.0	4.3	7.5	5.2	0.0	8.0	8.0	10.0	10.0	8.0	8.0
FMF HIV/AIDS	0.0	0.0	2.0	1.5	2.0	2.0	1.6	1.0	0.0	0.0	0.0	0.0	0.0
HIV/AIDS Subtotal	602.6	834.9	1103.5	1643.4	2263.4	2653.7	3699.2	5028.0	5487.6	5573.6	5439.5	5082.5	4544.1
USAID TB (CSH/GHCS/GHP)	50.0	60.0	64.2	74.7	79.4	79.2	80.8	148.0	162.5	225.0	224.6	236.0	224.0
USAID TB Other	12.0	12.0	12.4	10.4	12.6	12.3	14.1	15.2	14.1	18.2	13.8	13.8	8.0
TB Subtotal[c]	62.0	72.0	76.6	85.1	92.0	91.5	94.9	163.2	176.6	243.2	238.4	249.8	232.0
USAID Malaria (CSH/GHCS/GHP)	55.0	66.0	65.4	79.9	90.8	102.0	248.0	347.2	382.5	585.0	618.8	650.0	619.0
USAID Malaria Other	0.0	0.0	0.0	0.0	0.0	0.0	0.0	2.4	2.5	0.0	0.0	0.0	0.0
CDC Malaria	13.0	13.0	12.6	9.2	9.1	9.0	8.9	8.7	9.4	9.4	9.4	9.3	9.4
Malaria Subtotal	68.0	79.0	78.0	89.1	99.9	111.0	256.9	358.3	394.4	594.4	628.2	659.3	628.4
State Global Fund	0.0	0.0	0.0	0.0	0.0	198.0	377.5	545.5	600.0	750.0	748.5	1300.0	1650.0
USAID Global Fund	100.0	50.0	248.4	397.6	248.0	247.5	247.5	0.0	100.0	0.0	0.0	0.0	0.0
HHS Global Fund	0.0	125.0	99.0	149.0	99.2	99.0	99.0	294.8	300.0	300.0	297.3	0.0	0.0
Global Fund Subtotal	100.0	175.0	347.4	546.6	347.2	544.5	724.0	840.3	1000.0	1050.0	1045.8	1300.0	1650.0
HIV/AIDS, TB, Malaria Total	832.6	1160.9	1605.5	2364.2	2802.5	3400.7	4775.0	6389.8	7058.6	7461.2	7351.9	7291.6	7054.5

CRS-41

Source: Compiled by CRS from appropriations legislation, congressional budget justifications, the President's budget request, and interviews with U.S. officials.

Notes: n/s means not specified. n/a means not applicable.

a. Foreign Military Financing (FMF) account; Centers for Disease Control and Prevention (CDC); National Institutes of Health (NIH); Department of Labor (DOL); Department of Defense (DOD); Department of Health and Human Services (HHS), Child Survival and Health (CSH), Global Health Programs (GHP), Global Health and Child Survival (GHCS), Global HIV/AIDS Initiative (GHAI).

b. This includes funding from the Development Assistance Account (DA), the Economic Support Fund Account (ESF), and the Assistance for Europe, Eurasia, and Central Asia Account (AEECA).

c. CDC does not receive appropriations for global TB programs specifically. Instead it spends portions of its TB budget on international programs.

Table C-2. FY2001-FY2012 Global HIV/AIDS, TB, and Malaria Funding Totals in Constant Dollars

(constant U.S. $ millions)

Disease/Program Totals	FY2001 Actual	FY2002 Actual	FY2003 Actual	FY2004 Actual	FY2005 Actual	FY2006 Actual	FY2007 Actual	FY2008 Actual	FY2009 Actual	FY2010 Actual	FY2011 Actual	FY2012 Estimate
HIV/AIDS	761.9	1041.5	1347.1	1956.1	2608.3	2959.6	4020.5	5274.7	5720.4	5706.3	5439.5	5082.5
TB	78.4	89.8	93.5	101.3	106.0	102.0	103.1	171.2	184.1	249.0	238.4	249.8
Malaria	86.0	98.5	95.2	106.1	115.1	123.8	279.2	375.9	411.1	608.6	628.2	659.3
Global Fund	126.4	218.3	424.1	650.6	400.1	607.3	786.9	881.5	1042.4	2075.0	1045.8	1300.0
HIV/AIDS, TB, Malaria Total	1052.6	1448.2	1959.9	2814.0	3229.6	3792.7	5189.8	6703.3	7358.1	7638.8	7351.9	7291.6

Source: Compiled by CRS from appropriations legislation and interviews with U.S. officials.

Notes: Calculations into constant dollars are made using the FY2011 estimate total non-defense deflator, from the U.S. Government Printing Office, "Budget of the United States Government: Historical Tables Fiscal Year 2013," available at http://www.whitehouse.gov/omb/budget/Historicals.

Appendix D. HIV/AIDS, Tuberculosis, and Malaria Program Maps

Two maps are shown for each disease. The first displays U.S. bilateral funding levels across countries. The second highlights U.S. countries receiving assistance in relation to global prevalence estimates for each disease.

HIV/AIDS

Figure D-1 shows U.S. bilateral HIV/AIDS funding levels across countries in FY2009. **Figure D-2** highlights U.S. countries receiving assistance in relation to global HIV prevalence estimates in 2009.

Tuberculosis

Figure D-3 shows U.S. bilateral TB funding levels across countries in FY2009. **Figure D-4** highlights U.S. countries receiving assistance in relation to global TB prevalence estimates in 2009.

Malaria

Figure D-5 shows U.S. bilateral malaria funding levels across countries in FY2009. **Figure D-6** highlights U.S. countries receiving assistance in relation to global malaria prevalence estimates in 2009.

Figure D-1. U.S. Bilateral HIV/AIDS Funding, by Country, FY2009

(current U.S. $ millions)

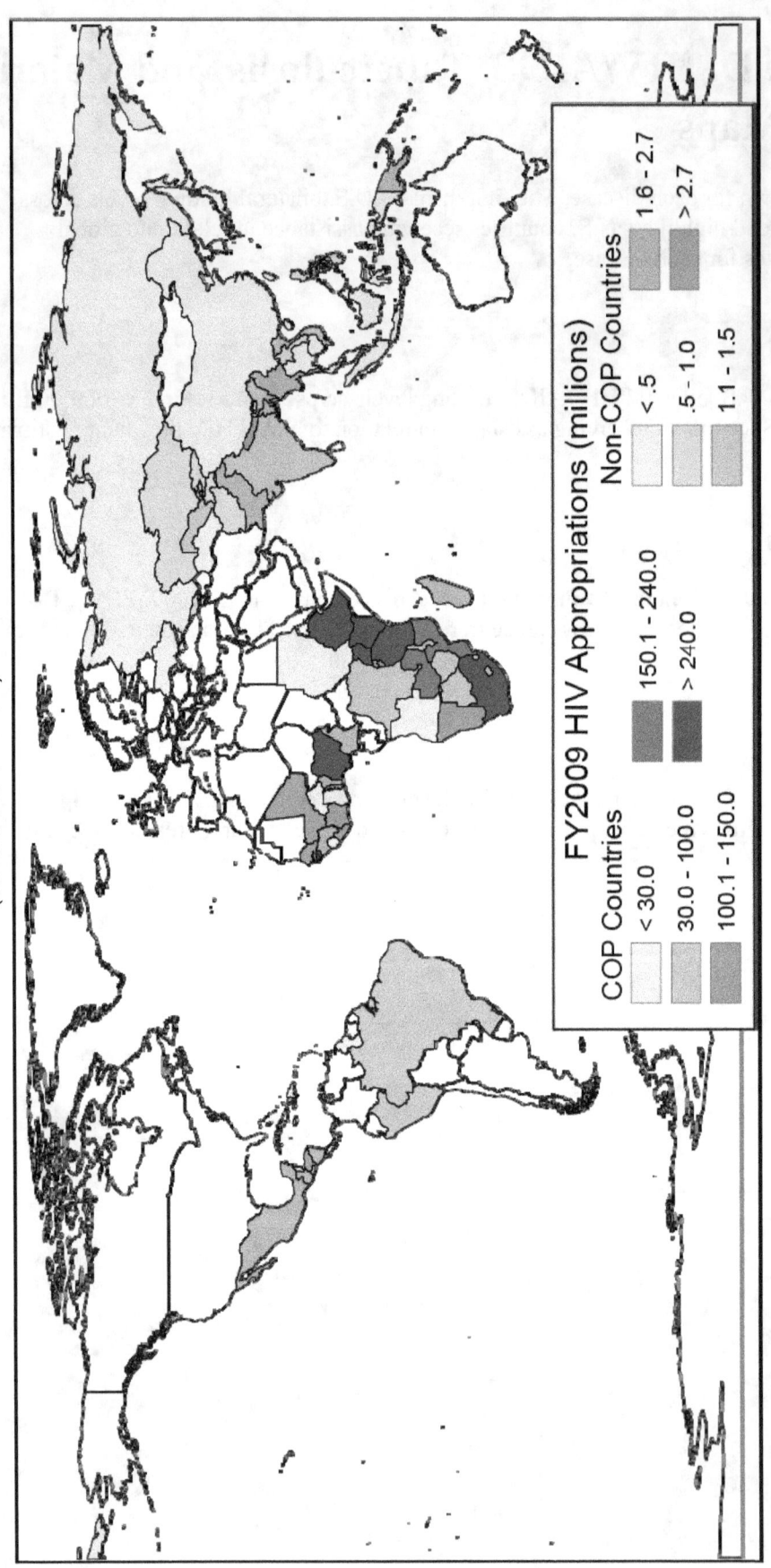

Source: Compiled by CRS from appropriations legislation and foreignassistance.gov.

Notes: COP countries refer to PEPFAR countries with "Country Operational Plans." COPs document U.S. annual investments and HIV/AIDS program targets, and serve as the basis for approval of annual U.S. bilateral HIV/AIDS funding to each country. A number of countries receiving smaller amounts of PEPFAR assistance are not required to submit COPs.

Figure D-2. HIV Prevalence Rates and PEPFAR COP Countries, 2009

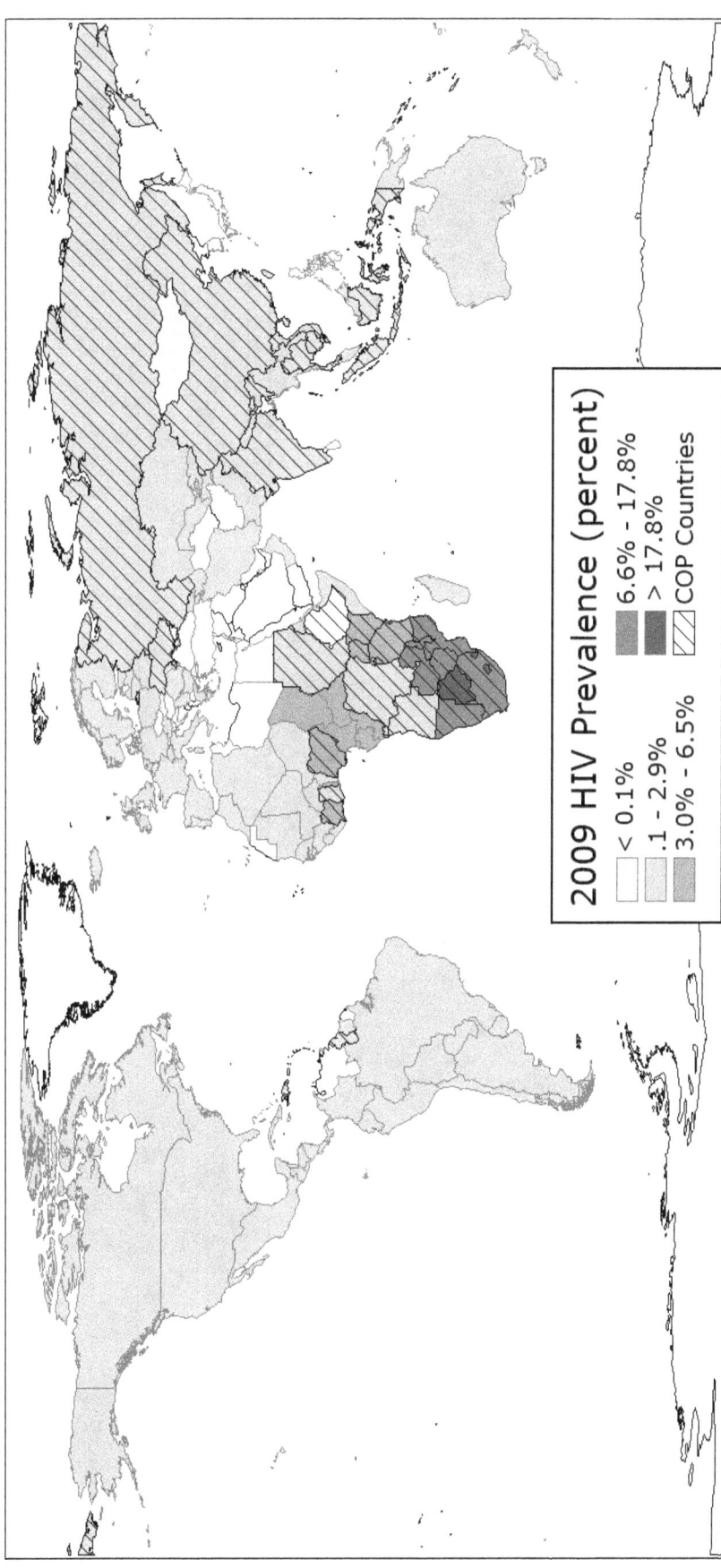

Source: Compiled by CRS from UNAIDS, *Report on the Global AIDS Epidemic,* 2010, http://www.unaids.org/globalreport/Global_report.htm, appropriations legislation, and foreignassistance.gov.

Notes: HIV prevalence measures the rate of infection among adults aged 5-49 in each country in 2009. COP countries refer to PEPFAR countries with "Country Operational Plans." COPs document U.S. annual investments and HIV/AIDS program targets, and serve as the basis for approval of annual U.S. bilateral HIV/AIDS funding to each country.

Figure D-3. U.S. Bilateral TB Funding, by Country, FY2009
(current U.S. $ millions)

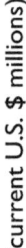

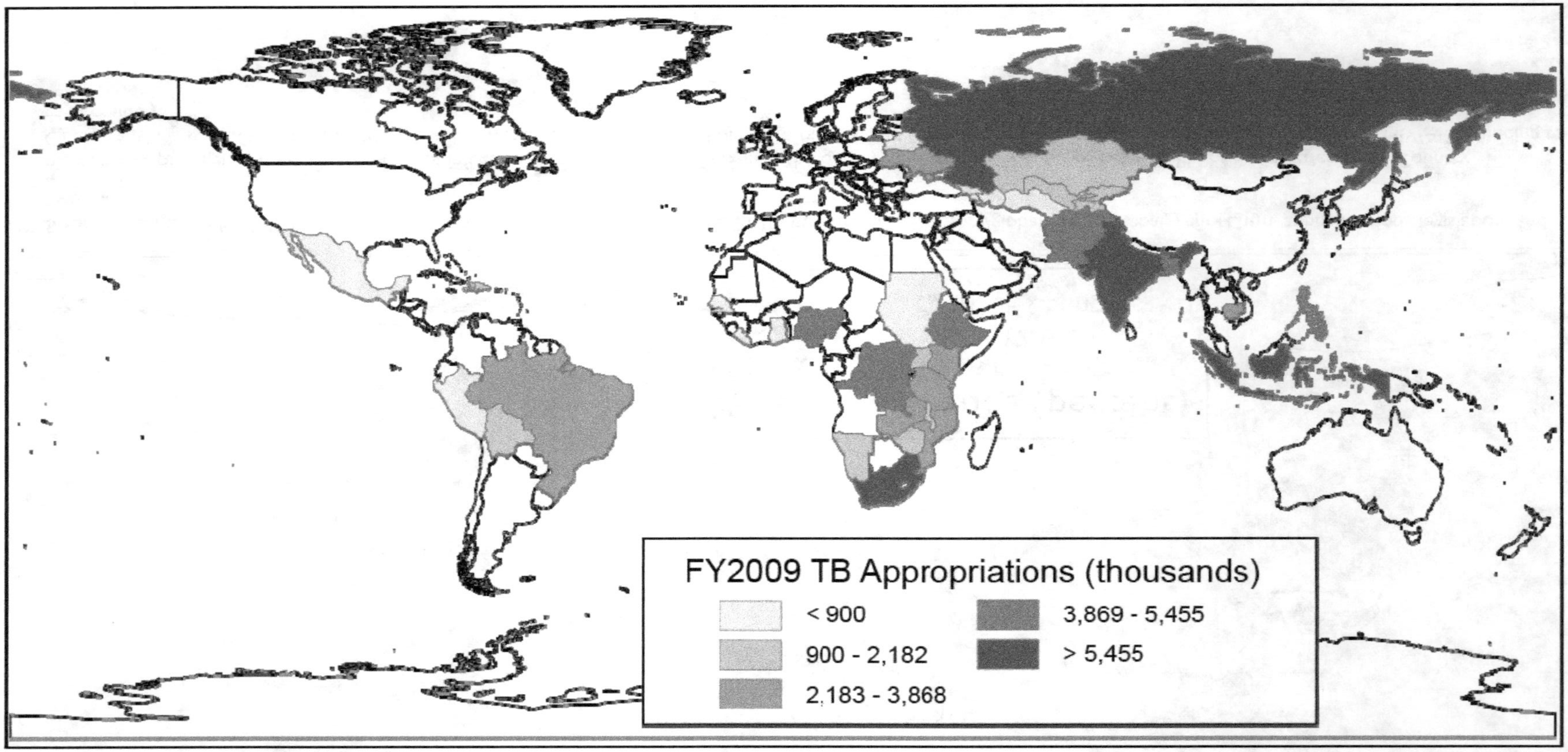

Source: Compiled by CRS from appropriations legislation and foreignassistance.gov.

Figure D-4. TB Prevalence Rates and USAID TB Countries, 2009

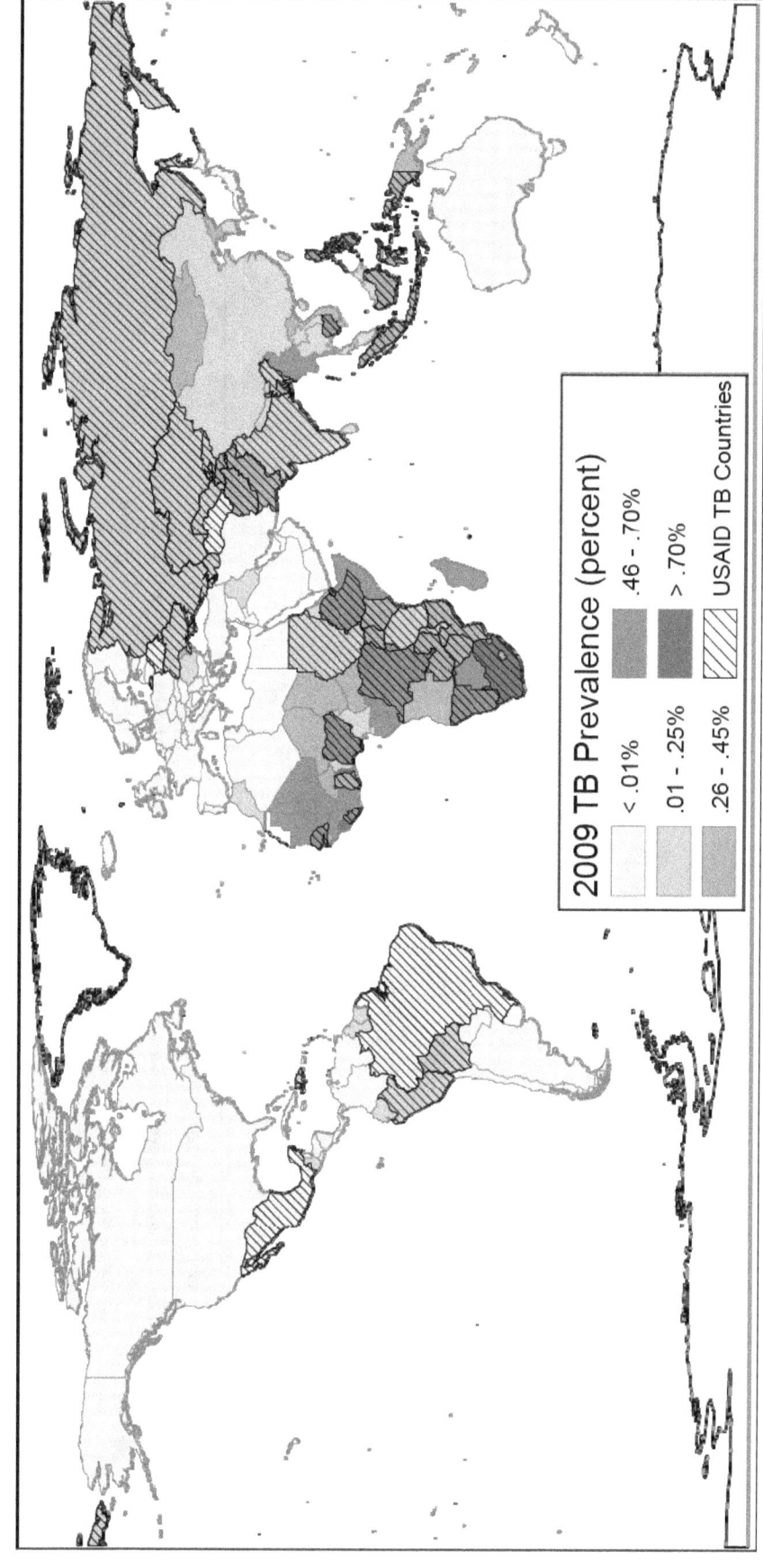

Source: Compiled by CRS from WHO, *Global Tuberculosis Control*, 2010, http://whqlibdoc.who.int/publications/2010/9789241564069_eng.pdf, appropriations legislation, and foreignassistance.gov.

Notes: TB prevalence measures the rate of infection in each country in 2009.

Figure D-5. U.S. Bilateral Malaria Funding, by Country, FY2009

(current U.S. $ millions)

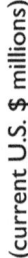

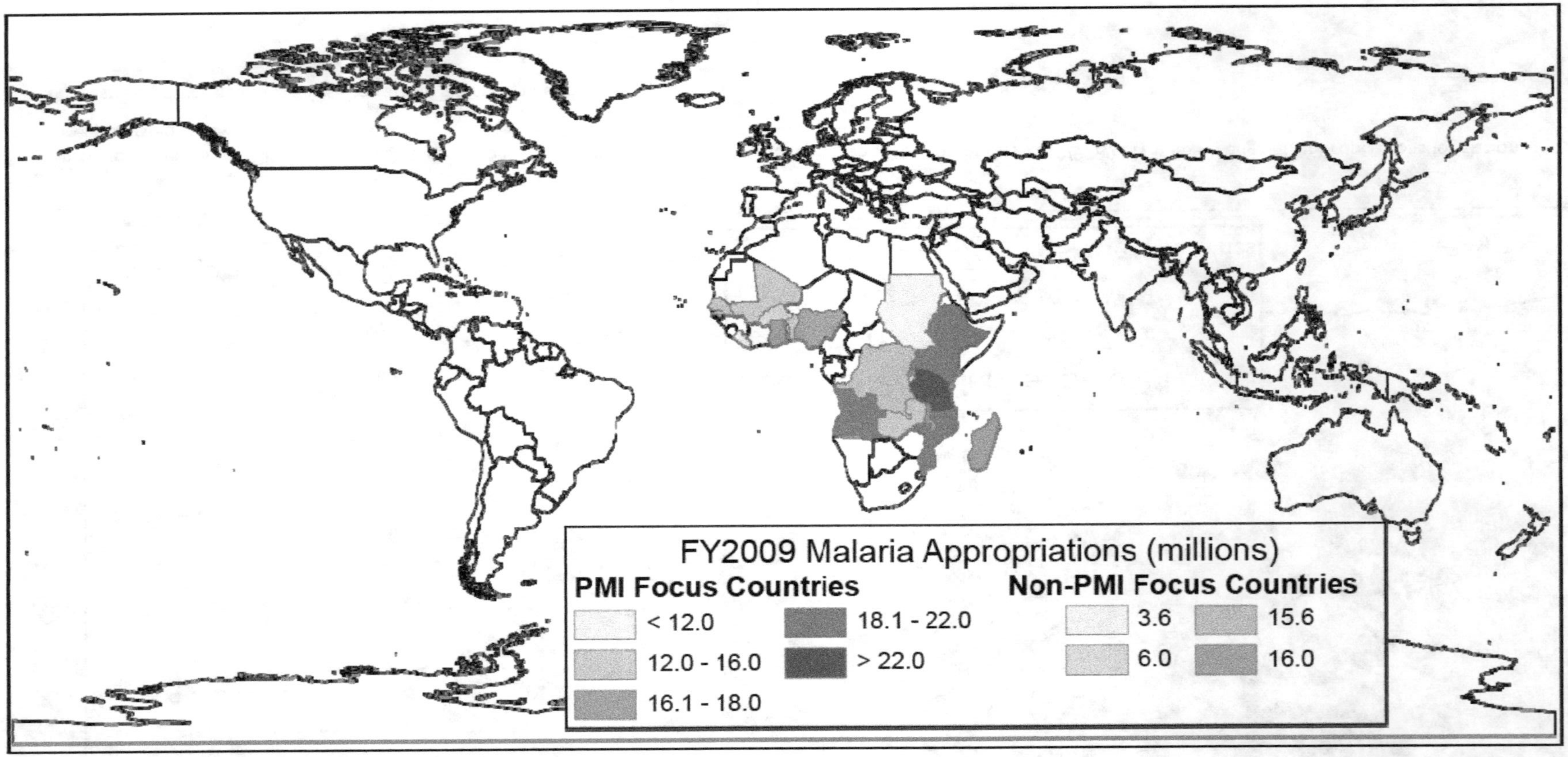

Source: Compiled by CRS from appropriations legislation and foreignassistance.gov.

Notes: In FY2009, PMI had 15 focus countries. Several other countries were receiving bilateral malaria assistance, but were not considered PMI focus countries.

Figure D-6. Malaria Prevalence Rates and PMI Focus Countries, 2009

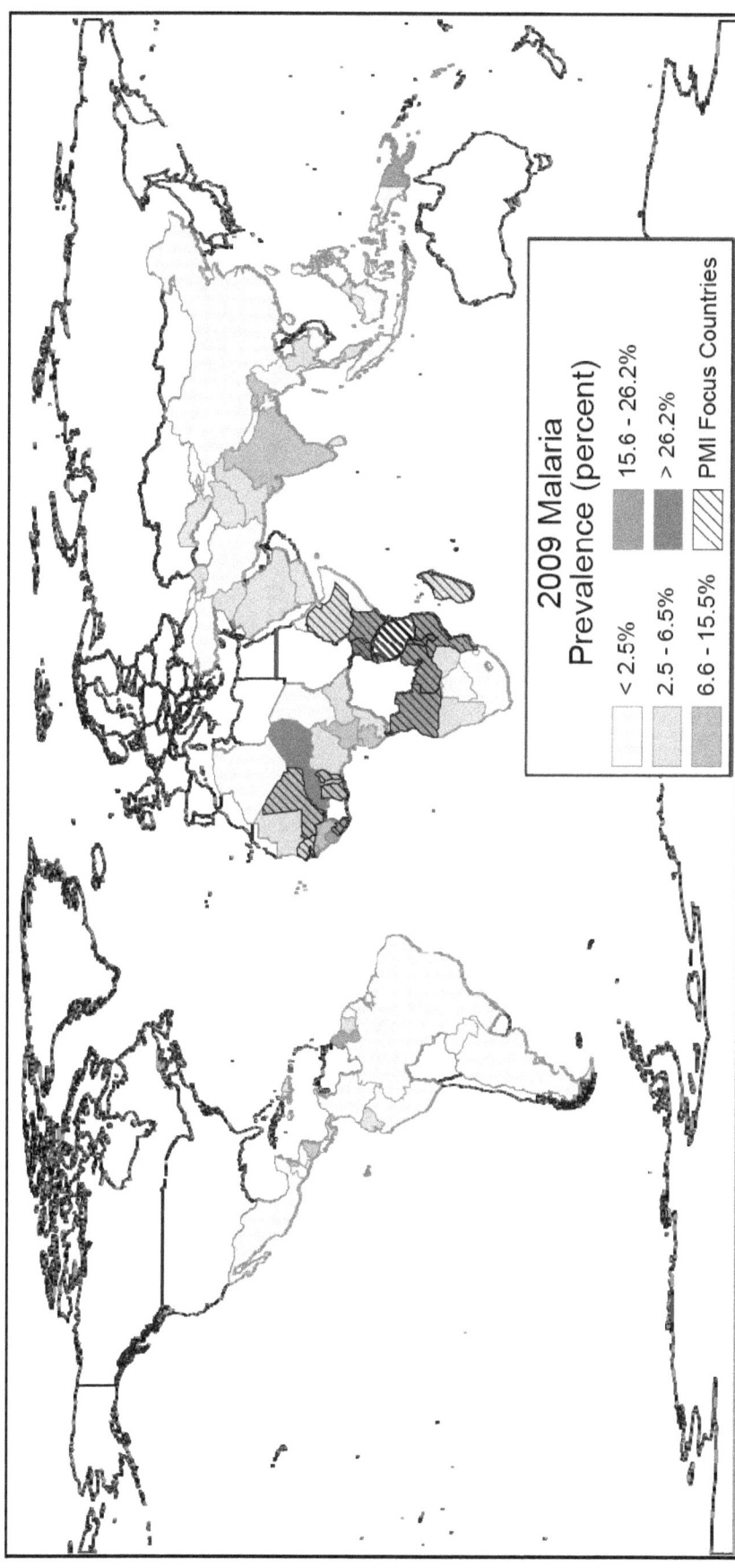

Source: Compiled by CRS from WHO, *World Malaria Report*, 2010, http://wholibdoc.who.int/publications/2010/9789241564106_eng.pdf, appropriations legislation, and foreignassistance.gov.

Notes: Malaria prevalence measures the rate of infection in each country in 2009.

Author Contact Information

Alexandra E. Kendall
Analyst in Global Health
akendall@crs.loc.gov, 7-7314

www.ingramcontent.com/pod-product-compliance
Lightning Source LLC
Chambersburg PA
CBHW081617170526
45166CB00009B/3007